"I was in a TV media-training seminar with Allan where we had to pitch in front of TV News Producers on Skype. It was just like Shark Tank except we had 3 minutes to pitch to twelve of the Executive Producers individually and we only had one shot to get on their station.

Allan helped me bring my energy up right before every pitch by doing very simple and power exercises. Best of all, it only took five minutes. With his help, I got booked on all 14 TV stations across the country!

Since then, I have also appeared on National syndicated shows like Doctor Oz, The Doctors, Bethenny, Daytime and many other TV news stations and before I get on the show, I would do exactly what Allan had taught me.

Whether you are a public speaker, sales person, executive or business owner, you need to read this book because your clients will be attracted to your awesome energy, aliveness and presence!"

— Dr. Kellyann Petrucci, M.S., N.D. Author of New York Times Best Seller Dr. Kellyann's Bone Broth Diet. She is a regular guest on The Doctors, Dr. Oz, and national news programs. DrKellyann.com

"Allan was recently on my Wellness for Life radio show and I am so excited that he has finally put his twelve years of research into print and helping millions alleviate stress, fatigue and insomnia. If you're suffer from adrenal burnout, you are tired all the time, you can't sleep at night, and you're overwhelmed with stress, then you will find long-lasting relief by implementing Allan's simple but powerful methods. Practicing his exercises consistently will up level your health to ultimate wellness for life!"

— Dr. Susanne Bennett Best selling author of The 7-Day Allergy Makeover and host of The Wellness for Life radio show on RadioMD & iHeart Radio DrSusanne.com

"Allan Ting in his new book has succinctly presented the case for how energy (positive and negative) dominates our lives. By following his simple and effective steps to recognize our energy level, shift our thinking patterns, and commit to daily movement and exercise rituals, we can significantly impact our health and wellbeing. Highly recommended reading."

— Dr. Cynthia Thaik Best selling author of Your Vibrant Heart: Restoring Health, Strength & Spirit from the Body's Core. DrCynthia.com

"As an OBGYN and a Hormone Expert in women's health, I see thousands of patients every year that suffer from work-related stress. Stress not only wreaks havoc in our immune system but is also one of the instant killers in intimacy. Allan was on my podcast as an expert interview recently and shared his heartbreaking story about how chronic stress affected his work and ultimately his intimate relationship. Through his heartbreak, he became inspired to seek out the best stress relieving methods. Now he condensed 10+ years all of his research, practice and teaching into this book. What he teaches is absolutely amazing and simple! He taught us this one simple cortisol (stress hormone) relieving exercises in our interview. In matter of minutes, my body felt lighter, I felt more grounded, more even more present. With the rich energy state, I am able to serve more clients and be more present with my family. As a physician and Hormone Expert, I understand why Allan's exercises changes our biochemistry when we move our body a certain way. However, you don't need to know how electricity works to turn on the light. Flip the switch by doing what Allan tells you and get ready to feel energized!"

— Dr. Anna Cabeca, DO, FACOG, ABAARM Cabecahealth.com

"Oh, wow. Finally a book on health and vitality that not only tells you what to do, but shows you how and explains exactly why, with honesty, wit and genuine caring. If you think you know all about vitality and energy but you aren't doing what you know, then read this book and change your life!"

— Mindy Gibbins-Klein Multi-award-winning entrepreneur, speaker and author MindyGK.com

The world's best speakers master their own energy because they know those with the most certainty and enthusiasm and those who serve from their hearts will electrify audiences and move them to action. In this book, Allan will teach you how to master your own magnetic energy right before your public appearance in five minutes! As founder of the Creative Performance Group, I created the Speakers Bootcamp, which is an intensive training that has created successful speakers, coaches, consultants and authors worldwide. The graduates of this program are making an impact in their lives and businesses because they can speak with confidence and purpose in any situation. Allan is a shining example of our family of graduates…not only as a teacher with wisdom and talent… but also as a person. His commitment to integrity and passion for helping people is amazing to see. He is truly a role model and someone who you should get to know. I encourage you to contact him through his website or Facebook… or even the old fashioned telephone… and see what he can do to transform your life!"

— Joe Williams, Strategic Expert Specializing in Creating World-Class Public Speaker JoeWilliamsOnline.com

"Allan Ting has done a masterful job of breaking down the necessary steps and mental understanding of how to reclaim your life by activating your energy and vitality through his Instant Energy Method. This is a must read book for beginners, intermediate and advanced practitioners who desire more focus, productivity and influence at work!"

— Hon. Micki I. Aronson Retired Federal Judge

"Allan Ting has found the Fountain Of Youth. Millions search for the Fountain all their lives and never find it. Well here is your map. If you want to live a longer, healthier, happier life, the secret is in your hands."

— Aaron Scott Young CEO Laughlin Associates, Inc laughlinusa.com

"When we experience chronic stress and low energy, our emotional intelligence and productivity diminishes. Through Allan's own personal struggle of poor health, low energy and near homelessness, he inspires us to take care of our own health and energy first. Because when we feel great and are full of energy, we radiate our authenticity and positive vibe everywhere. That is when we become even more influential to the people around us."

— Mike Robbins Author of Nothing Changes Until You Do, Mike-Robbins.com

"Allan is one of our yoga teachers at Yahoo. He is not only a great yoga teacher, but also an inspiring mentor for being a better person. Attending his lesson has been one of my weekly priorities no matter how busy I am at work. I used to have back pain and felt stressed about work very often; however, my overall physical and mental health have improved a lot after following his advice. His positive energy and attitude make his class very popular. From time to time, it is difficult to secure a space if you don't show up early enough. I am so happy he compiled the practical skills he shared with us in this book. I highly recommend his book to anyone who is struggling to live a happy and healthy life."

— Changming Yang Director, Search Editorial at Yahoo!

"Allan Ting's Instant Energy Method delivers the boost to get access to energy, instantly. In his three step POW Process, you get the lesson – and reminder – you need to step it up in any situation. He then teaches us how to eliminate the elements in our lives that sap our energy. And finally, he gives us some super tools to keep us charged. At the end of each section are high performance questions to ensure we know where we're going! Allan gives us plenty of stories, plenty of exercises, plenty of references to back up his advice. I feel better having just read the book. Now to stretch!"

— Dr Wayne Pernell High Performance Leadership Coach
DynamicLeader.com

"This book will motivate you to take stock of what is most important to your success and personal fulfillment. If you want more energy or simply or want to know more about how energy works, Allan Ting's book, Instant Energy Method is a must read!"

— Marlene Chism Author of No-Drama Leadership MarleneChism.com

"Allan Ting has a deep understanding and clear perspective of what it takes to live a vibrant and productive life. He shares expertise drawn from his personal journey and the best of ancient practices and modern science to help you learn how to experience genuine vitality. He provides practical strategies that are easy to follow and apply. Make the choice now to continuously enjoy and live daily from an energy rich state. It's the right time to put into action this must read energy guide!"

— Joan I. Rosenberg, PhD Author of Ease Your Anxiety and Mean Girls,
Meaner Woman DrJoanRosenberg.com

"It's about time this book was written. It is a long-overdue guide for the new generation of high achievers who desire a more meaningful and relevant lifestyle, and Allan Ting is the ideal ambassador. This will be huge."

— Chef Mark Garcia Best selling author and founder of Rock Star Chef
Marketing Academy ChefMarkGarcia.com

"Allan Ting is an Elite ENERGY Coach who will challenge you to be more strategic about your mindset and management of energy. He has a compelling story, a readable synthesis of the latest research and coaches you with competence, humor and deep caring. Alan has clearly been influenced by master teachers and has developed his own simplified and innovative method to help you notice your own self-technology and amplify energy. You'll feel his method working quickly and will experience new levels of balance, stamina and vibrancy that you just knew were lying latent in yourself all along. Enjoy!"

— Michelle Vendelin, Founder, Silicon Valley High Performance
SVHighPerformance.com

"What a great book to learn how to easily boost energy fast in a very mentally and physically healthy way. I love the simple POW awareness, because it is so easy to remember. I also love the part about how to quickly reduce belly fat in 4 days! The part explains the effect of coffee really got my attention! I will use EFT to imprint in my mind so that I don't fall into the coffee trap again. In conclusion, I must say, if you want to naturally carrying abundant positive energy, follow the simple exercises in this book. It won't take more than a week before you can feel the magical difference! Namaste."

— Carol Lin Transformational Energy Psychology Therapist, High Performance Coach, Published Author, and Speaker. Emlmcoach.com

"Time is a finite resource, but the energy that wells up within us is quite renewable. Using his gift of storytelling and his knack for practical, instant application, Allan Ting expounds upon the scientific research on energy management, so that anyone from a casual reader to a Zen master can implement tips and obtain internal rewards of renewed energy immediately. He has produced a great read, something I wish I'd have had available to me thirty years ago!"

— Scott Carbonara (aka, The Leadership Therapist) Bestselling author of Manager's Guide to Employee Engagement LeadershipTherapist.com

"This fabulous book is for anyone who wants more energy — and who doesn't want more energy? Allan Ting has written the handbook for instantly boosting your energy as well as increasing a sustained level of energy for the long run. As someone who has suffered from chronic stress and fatigue—and effectively managed himself through it, he can personally relate to all the symptoms and painful results from being overwhelmed, overweight, burnt out and sleep deprived, which seems to be a national epidemic. Allan provides simple, practical tips that you can implement immediately, steps you can take to achieve lasting improvement, and great depth of knowledge about what drains our energy and what to do about it. He combines his personal experience with the study he made of all the great practices, including Yoga, Meditation, Tai Chi and Qigong and his in depth knowledge of Neuroscience and NLP. It's a winning combination. You can sense his energy and passion for this topic as you read, resulting in the personal motivation to take the steps that will make the difference. Put this book on your reading list and make it a priority—you'll be glad you did!"

— Cheryl Bonini Ellis Author, Speaker, Trainer and Coach on High Performance and Leadership Excellence EllisBusinessEnterprises.com

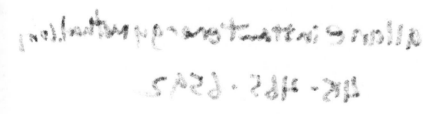

Dear Jennifer,

POW!

To your success,

[signature]

allan@instantenergymethod.com
415-465-6592

The Instant Energy Method™

3 Secret Hacks to Boost Your Focus,
Productivity and Influence at Work

Allan Ting

Copyright © 2016 Allan Ting and My Yoga Stream Corp.

All Rights Reserved. No part of this publication may be reproduced or transmitted in any form or by any means, mechanical or electronic, including photocopying and recording, or by any information storage and retrieval system, without permission in writing from the author or publisher (except by a reviewer, who may quote brief passages and/or show brief video clips in a review).

Disclaimer: The Publisher and the Author make no representation or warranties with respect to the accuracy or completeness of the contents of this work and specifically disclaim all warranties of fitness for a particular purpose. No warranty may be created or extended by sales or promotional materials. The advice and strategies contained herein may not be suitable for every situation. This work is sold with the understanding that the Publisher is not engaged in rendering legal, accounting or other professional services. If professional assistance is required, the services of a competent professional person should be sought. Neither the Publisher nor the Author shall be liable for damages arising therefrom. The fact that an organization or website is referred to in this work as citation and/or potential source of further information does not mean that the Author or the Publisher endorses the information, the organization or website may provide or recommendations it may make. Further, readers should be aware that internet websites listed in this work may have changed or disappeared between when this work was written and when it is read.

This book is not intended as a substitute for the medical advice of physicians. The reader should regularly consult a physician in matters relating to his/her health and particularly with respect to any symptoms that may require diagnosis or medical attention. The authors and publisher advise readers to take full responsibility for their safety and know their limits. Before practicing the skills described in this book, be sure that your equipment is well maintained, and do not take risks beyond your level of experience, aptitude, training, and comfort level.

First Edition 2016

Printed in the United States of America

Cover Design by: Allan Ting

Published by:
My Yoga Stream Corp
PO Box 2401
Rocklin, CA 95677
www.AllanTing.com

For more information about Allan Ting or to book him for your next event, speaking engagement, podcast or media interview please visit: www.AllanTing.com

Dedication

This book is dedicated to those of us who struggle with work related stress, fatigue and low energy. May this book help you find your own happiness, inner peace, and serenity.

I want to take a moment and dedicate this book to my wife for your never-ending encouragements 加油 (add gas) which refuel my passion in life.

To my daughter, Siena, English is your dad's second language; he didn't learn how to speak English until the age of eight. His fourth grade English teacher thought he was mentally deranged, so she sent him to see a child psychiatrist. His tenth grade English teacher stood him beside her podium and lectured him for ten minutes as she drew across his five-page term paper with red lines, circles, arrows, and scribbles—and announced to everyone in the class what a horrible writer he was. His freshman English professor in college wanted to fail him, so that he would retake English 114.

There will be days when you want to give up, but do the best with what you have. Love and serve the world from your heart.

Let your own light shine.

Don't ever let anybody tell you otherwise.

Love,

Dad

Acknowledgments

Thank you Mom and Dad for believing in me—and supporting me along this journey and in my passion.

Thank you Laura Steward for your mentoring, inspiration, and helping me believe that I need to share my story with the world.

Thank you Jocelyn Godfrey for all of your great feedback and encouragements.

Last, thank you Gil Bardsley for your English tutoring in college helping me find my voice and your encouraging words of, "Wow, Allan, you know how to write. I didn't know they taught writing in public schools!" Your words forever live in my heart.

Table of Contents

Your Surprise Bonus...xix

Foreword..1

Preface...5

Energy – What is it and why do we all need it?.........................5

Introduction...21

The Four Energy Quadrants:

Quadrant 1:   Energy Rich, Energy Lasting State....................27

Quadrant 2:   Energy Rich, Energy Non-Lasting State..........28

Quadrant 3:   Energy Poor, Exhaustion State.........................29

Quadrant 4:   Energy Poor, Lethargic State............................30

What Not to Do..31

How to Get the Most Out of This Book.................................35

Best of Both Worlds – Ancient Practice

Meets Modern Science...37

Secret Energy Hack Section I — Jump Start Your
Own Energy Naturally...39

Overview 41

Chapter 1:   First Energy Booster: Watch Your Posture......47

Chapter 2:   Second Energy Booster: Oxygenate

Your Body 51

Chapter 3: Third Energy Booster: Water 57

Chapter 4: How and When Do You Use the Abundance
Energy Exercises to Help Yourself to Stay on
Top of Your Game? 61

Action Step Exercises 64

Section I — Game Changer Questions 65

**Secret Energy Hack Section II — What Drains
Our Life Energy?** 67

Overview 69

Chapter 5: Diet Intake 73

Chapter 6: Release Stress 75

Chapter 7: Activity and Non-Movement 79

Chapter 8: Identify Toxins 83

Chapter 9: Negative Language Patterns 93

Action Step Exercises 100

Section II — Game Changer Questions 101

**Secret Energy Hack Section III — Manage Your
Energy for Life** 103

Overview 105

Chapter 10: Qigong – The 2,000-year-old Ancient
Secret Energy Practice 109

Action Step Exercises 116

Chapter 11: Top 7 Natural Foods to Sustain Your
Quadrant 1, Energy Rich Energy Lasting
State 117

Section III — Game Changer Questions 128

Secret Energy Hack Section IV – Advance Energy State: The Joy of Pure Energy 129

Overview 131

Chapter 12: The Gin and Juice of Neuroscience Alchemy: SIP (Somatosensory, Insula, Prefrontal Cortex) 143

Action Step Exercises...151

Chapter 13: Mind and Body Connection 153

Action Step Exercises...163

Chapter 14: The Science of Being Thankful and Grateful 165

Chapter 15: Emotional Detox and Cleansing Through Sound and Vibrations 171

Action Step Exercises...174

Section IV — Game Changer Questions...........................175

Putting It All Together 177

Epilogue..179

References 189

About the Author...195

Your Surprise Bonus

This book is not meant for you to read passively while you're lying on your bed eating biscuit with milk. I hope I got you laughing. Rather it's an interactive experience that has been carefully designed to help you take your focus, productivity, and influence at work to the next level and most importantly, having fun going through the process.

To assist in this, I have created an interactive pictorial workbook that will walk you through step-by-step exercises on creating your own abundant energy. This book will give you the context to understand why we do the exercises in the workbook and the workbook will help you get results with ease.

As my gift to you, I am including the interactive workbook as a part of Instant Energy Method™ book.

Download Your Complimentary Workbook at www.AllanTing.com/IEMBookBonuses

Foreword

As a naturopathic medical doctor with a thyroid-focused practice, my schedule is tight. In addition to running my clinic, I also write books and share my advice on national television across the country.

I need to have top energy for my work and also so I can show my full presence and love for my wonderful wife and two kids. Family is my biggest priority. I am one of those doctors who practice what he preaches. I watch what I eat—and avoid coffee and sugar. I am an avid athlete and love running, rock climbing, and biking of all types. So before meeting Allan, my health and energy levels were already high.

Then something happened...

I was lucky enough to spend a week in the Caribbean with Allan and do his energy sessions each morning. After each session, I saw firsthand how my energy boosted to a whole new level that I didn't even know existed. I was hooked!

I found his simple and gentle energy sequences—regulating the body's vital energy—to be very powerful. I had taken yoga and meditation classes before, but I discovered that what Allan teaches is something truly unique, insightful, and completely inspiring.

For the next six days, I attended his "Hour of Power" classes every morning. I found that I was consistently in a better mood after these mind-body therapy sessions.

Why was this important for my everyday life?

I am always eager to gain the extra edge that will help my doctors, nurses, administrative staff, and myself help people more effectively.

Whether you run your own business working long hours, or you work for a company and want to get promoted and recognized, having even more energy will help you reach the next level.

I love what Allan taught so much that I brought his simple and powerful exercises back to my workplace after the retreat. We projected Allan's Instant Energy Method videos onto a big screen, and my staff and I did his simple energy exercises in the mornings to boost everyone's energy levels. The exercises helped us pick up our energy levels, set the tone of the day, and provide long lasting energy— as we increased our circulation of good energy and cleansed our body of negative energy. The best part about the exercises is they only took five minutes—and we all had so much fun doing them!

Allan's practice is so important in my line of work. I have an extremely high standard when it comes to patient care, because many patients come to my clinic as a "last chance effort." Patients' lives are in our hands, and we do our best to restore their health and lives back to order—which means we need to be in the best physical and mental state possible to facilitate their progress.

I find that when I gain more energy, it overflows to every part of my day. My mood throughout the day is phenomenal, because I have great energy to feed it. Simply put, by taking care of ourselves at the clinic, we take great care of patients. The doctors and the nurses feel it. Our administration staffs feel it. Our patients feel it—and return the positive energy back to us.

Our staff works better, and it overflows to how we interact with people. Our patients respond back to us with great energy too. Because of this, my staff and I *thrive* at work.

Allan's program has been phenomenal and incredible to this process. The only way I can describe his teaching is the "Allan Ting Method," as he blends a 2,000-year-old ancient practice into one that supports a modern, busy life. This is something you truly need to experience yourself—as others are. It wasn't until later that I learned that Allan had already been teaching his Instant Energy Method at large tech companies like Yahoo, eBay, Amazon, and at Tony Robbins live seminars.

I am honored and grateful to be a part of Allan's book, because the man truly cares and serves from his heart. His personal story of struggle—from not being able to get out of bed with chronic stress and fatigue for over six months, to his success today—is exceptionally inspirational.

Now he shares his simple and powerful step-by-step routines to help us have more abundant energy in our lives. We know firsthand that when we lose our health and vitality, our livelihood suffers. Our career, love life, finances, family, and kids all get jeopardized with low energy.

Energy and health create the baseline of our success in life. If we master vitality, we can overcome any challenges that come into our lives—and create the wealth that we deserve.

Allan's Instant Energy Method is remarkable; but don't just take my word for it. Start reading his book, and find out for yourself how simple it is have even more focus, productivity, and influence at work. You'll feel great, have long lasting energy, and may even look younger—if you do what Allan says!

Ready for the challenge?!?

—Alan Christianson, NMD Author of New York Times Best Seller,
The Adrenal Reset Diet

Alan Christianson, NMD, is one of the foremost authorities on thyroid and adrenal disorders. He founded Integrative Health, a physician group dedicated to helping people with thyroid disease and weight loss resistance regain their health. Named a Top Doctor in Phoenix magazine, he has been featured on numerous publications and has been on The Doctors, Dr. Oz, CNN and Today show. He trains other physicians in the U.S. and internationally on management of thyroid disease, weight loss and hormone replacement. He is the author of the New York Times Best Seller, The Adrenal Reset Diet, the Complete Idiot's Guide to Thyroid Disease, and Healing Hashimoto's – a Savvy Patient's Guide. Integrativehealthcare.com

Preface

The Dalai Lama, when asked what surprised him most about humanity, answered, *"Man... Because he sacrifices his health in order to make money. Then he sacrifices money to recuperate his health. And then is so anxious about the future that he does not enjoy the present; the result being that he does not live in the present or the future; he lives as if he is never going to die, and then dies having never really lived."*

Energy – What is it and why do we all need it?

We all need energy to jump out of bed and get our days going. Whether it is working hard so that we can get a raise and a promotion, successfully running our own business, or being the best husband or wife or dad or mom—whatever our aspiration is—we must have energy to fuel our passion in life.

Some manage their energy state better than others, but eventually even the most successful people experience burnout—at least some time in their lives. It took Arianna Huffington, one of the most successful and influential women in the world, lying in her pool of blood with a broken cheekbone and five stitches underneath her eyebrows, to realize that she was exhausted, sleep deprived, and burnt out from work. It was an awakening for her to redefine what success was. She self reflected to reprioritize what was important in her life—and how to get the most from her health, wisdom, joy, and giving.

In our modern society, only a select handful of people live in the *energy rich state.* The *"energy rich state"* occurs when we experience the highest levels of joy, presence, vitality, and gratitude on a consistent basis. The people in this category don't feel this just one day. They have been living at this level of life for decades.

For the rest of us, we barely touch the rim of the energy rich state. We try to get there by fueling ourselves with caffeinated beverages to help us get going in the morning. Without coffee, we default back into an *energy poor state:* groggy and sluggish. We need our coffee, or otherwise we walk around like zombies from the TV series, *The Walking Dead.*

We also are living in one of the busiest times in human history. As the use of microchips, the Internet, and smartphones grow at an ultra-exponential pace, we also are wrapped in the growth frenzy on a more personal level as well. Many of us are putting more hours into work than we ever have. When I work with corporate executives and management teams at well-known tech companies, I often hear this question repeated over and over: "How do we do more with less?"

It's no wonder that the American Psychological Association reported a study on workplace stress, where 69 percent of employees reported that work is a significant source of stress and 41 percent expressed that they feel tense or stressed out during the work day. And 51 percent of employees said that they are less productive at work as a result of stress. In addition, 52 percent of employees thought about leaving their jobs because of work related stress.

Here is another interesting report. Accenture studied 4,100 business executives from medium to large companies across thirty-three countries and found this:

- 75 percent of the executives said that they work frequently or occasionally during paid time off—generally checking email, catching up on work, working with no distraction, and participating in conference calls.
- 40 percent considered themselves workaholics.

That's almost one in every two people working all the time. We are handcuffed to our phones—constantly checking emails and trying to check off one more task from our work lists. In fact, work almost *expects* us to be on top of email, even at 11:30 p.m. at night. If we aren't, we won't be able to catch up later, since that many more emails and requests will have come in. In addition, our colleagues and clients are expecting us to get back to them as soon as possible. Hence the traditional twenty-four hour email response time is now diminished to a two hour expectation as we live in a "go, go, go" and instant response life.

To cope with our fast paced lives, we need more energy to keep us going, day in and day out. So what do we do? How do we get our bodies into functional mode? How do we prepare ourselves for a busy day?

Historically, we've turned to quick fixes. We go for the caffeinated beverages. Have you ever noticed that there is a Starbucks on every corner in the metropolitan city with long lines at seven in the morning and four in the afternoon? Did you know that Starbucks made $16.4 billion in annual revenue in 2014? And Starbucks' revenue has been increasing steadily by 10 percent, year over year.

What about the little bottle with a red cap on top called the "5 Hour Energy Drink," sitting right in front of the cashier at your local convenient store? That little bottle also constitutes a billion dollar industry. That's not even accounting for all of the other brands of energy drinks.

People are looking to supplement lost energy, but we are turning to counterproductive, or at best, Band-Aid solutions.

You may say, "I love the taste of my venti latte, extra foam, extra hot with twenty shots of espresso." I get it. I'm not telling you to quit coffee. I, too, drank three cups of mocha with two shots of espresso a day. When I stopped drinking coffee, I felt like crap, which caused me to spiral further into my chronic fatigue.

Actually, I'm not telling you to quit coffee. But if you want to know why drinking coffee is one of the worst strategies to get more energy in your life, and how it may even be leeching your bone density, causing osteoporosis, we'll cover that topic more in the book.

In the end, coffee or energy drinks aren't what we are really after, are they? Isn't the byproduct what we want: getting more energy so that we have more focus and effectiveness at work?

Would you want to pay $32 per gallon for gasoline to run your car? No, of course not, but that is how much a gallon of grande latte cost. Our nation went on a fuel strike a few years ago when gasoline went over $4 a gallon, but we're glad to fork over $1,100 a year on Starbucks.

And this energy poor state further perpetuates into our well-being. It cuts in even in our sleep. The Center for Disease Control published an article in January 2014 headlined, "Inefficient Sleep Is a Public Health Epidemic." An estimated fifty million to seventy million adults in the US experience a *sleep wakefulness disorder.*

Why the epidemic? One of the leading culprits behind this sleep epidemic is day-to-day stress. Many of us lie in bed at night thinking about our work, our emails, and all of our "to-do lists." Then in the morning, we wake up feeling groggy, barely keeping our heads above water as we just try to survive the day. This is a vicious cycle that happens day in and day out.

How do lack of sleep and stress affect our lives? Studies have shown that long-term stress and lack of sleep (occurring over six or more months) contribute to many of the most common conditions such as heart diseases, diabetes, and an inability to lose weight. In one way or another, 99 percent of diseases can be traced back to stress.

This stress cycle is only getting worse. On March 7, 2013, the front page of USA Today reported that eight out of ten Americans are *"always working"* (Petrecca and Snider). The reason is because we have these new devices called smartphones—iPhone or Android—and we are connected online 24/7. Because we are tethered to the phone 24/7, many of us feel like we have to reply to our work emails.

If you don't believe me, let me ask you this. I'd like you to imagine for a moment that someone took your smartphone away from you for two days. That means you would have no access to the Internet, no Facebook connection, no Tweeting, and no email. Oh, by the way, you can't access your computer or other people's devices. How would you feel? Would you feel like you were in withdrawals? Would you feel naked? Would you feel like you had an urge to check your email? Would you feel FOMO (fear of missing out) with your Facebook friends posting silly cat videos? You may also experience phantom vibration, where you would reach for your phone in your pocket thinking you got a message, when there was nothing in your pocket. If you answered yes to any of these questions, you may have an addiction to your phone. You may laugh! I know; I have experienced it too! I mean have you ever felt obliged to reply to a work related email at 11 p.m. at night or even on the weekends? I know I have many times.

Psychologists call this the *Zeigarnik Effect*, when we remember uncompleted tasks rather than the ones we already finished. Hollywood knows this well, and that's why the most popular TV series like *House of Cards* with Kevin Spacey makes you want to watch the next episode season after season. It's like the itch that we just can't scratch. Unfortunately, work email is the same way, because when we finally catch up with the hundreds of emails at night, rest assured that there will be hundreds more when we wake up. It's no wonder why we are stressed out more than ever from work, because we are always working, and we don't get a chance to rest.

Work related stress causes employees to take time off from work, which also affects the employer's bottom line. *The Huffington Post* published an article stating that employees' missed work due to health problems is costing the US $84 billion each year. In addition, the research found that out of the 94,000 interviews conducted in 2012, 77 percent of US employees who work thirty hours or more a week were either overweight or obese, or had at least one chronic health condition. The worst health job types included business owners, executives, service workers, teachers, nurses, doctors, foresters, and transportation workers; these have the worst health (*Healthy Living Blog*, May 7, 2013).

You're probably thinking, "Yeah yeah, enough with the stats. Why are you telling me all of these things?" My point to you is this. Like with the national obesity epidemic wherein more than 50 percent of us are overweight, chronic stress and fatigue are also climbing the epidemic chart at an unprecedented rate. Stress and obesity go hand in hand.

I also know these statistics and findings well, because I was among them. In 2001, I suffered from chronic stress, chronic fatigue, and obesity. No matter how much I slept, I would still wake up feeling beyond tired. I would sleep about twelve to fourteen hour days just to wake up feeling groggy with low energy. I was in bed for more than six months. I felt really depressed and didn't want to do anything but go back to bed. I was stuck in a vicious cycle. My life fell apart. My girlfriend left me. I had no job and was one step away from homeless. I was also fifty pounds heavier than I am today. Yes, I was really fat! And on top of that, I had the added weight of supporting my retired mom and dad. I had to figure out how to do this, but I felt tired all the time, and I just didn't have any motivation. Oh, and my doctors—they couldn't do anything for me.

It took me six months of lying in bed to realize this simple concept: when we have low energy, it affects all aspects of our lives—whether with our careers, relationships, livelihood, or even financial situations. So I said to myself, "If I'm ever going to get out of this bed alive and experience my life, I need to heal myself naturally." I was determined to find a solution. Thus I began my quest to learn about energy.

I wanted to have more energy in my life, so I decided to get back into shape. I started bicycling, running, kickboxing—everything that boosted my energy state. But I was on this yo-yo energy spike, wherein I felt great for a moment, and then my energy level would plummet back down again. I still felt chronic fatigue and couldn't shake it off. I changed my diet to full vegan and cut out sugar and simple carbohydrates for over six months. Again, my energy level went up and down.

One Saturday morning as I was riding my mountain bike in Golden Gate Park, I saw a group of people doing tai chi as their morning exercise. I became really curious. I'd seen them do tai chi for many years. I just never bothered to stop and ask them how to start the practice—mostly because when I was a kid, I used to make fun of old Chinese people moving so slowly. The pace was way too slow, and besides, it looked really boring.

But on this day, I decided to stop and ask one of the tai chi teachers how to participate. She answered, "Well you know, just come every Saturday and Sunday. Our classes are held at eight o'clock. We do the full set of tai chi in the beginning, and afterwards, we have a breakout session for a different group."

Even though I thought it was hilarious to be stuck with seventy- to eighty-year-old grandmas and grandpas, I went anyway and dragged my dad with me. *Maybe they knew something that I didn't,* I thought.

Ironically, after the first session, I felt really energized. It was more of a workout than I had expected. The exercises looked simple and easy on the outside, but squatting and holding my arms up for hours took a lot of effort. The amazing thing was, I felt my body was more expanded and open. Despite being tired, I had more energy afterwards. So I was addicted, and I went back over and over.

Thus I started my twelve year journey of studying how to effectively reach toward the energy rich state in our busy everyday lives. The only challenge I found is that the tai chi sets would take over one-and-a-half hours to complete. So, I asked the question, *"How could we get more energy within a shorter amount of time, so that we could still function throughout the day—especially when we get to work?"* I was looking for answers.

A short time later in 2002, I found a job at a fast growing, high-tech company. I'd never had any account management experience, so I had to be on my A-game. If I was lethargic or tired all of the time, I would not be able to function at work or meet my key performance metrics. That also meant I'd be fired. And if I was fired, then I wouldn't be supporting my mom and dad, and I'd be on the street. In effect, I was *one step from being homeless.*

I continued to study tai chi on the weekends. Meanwhile, one Thursday afternoon while I was returning home from work, I got rear-ended by a U-Haul truck that had run a red light. This injury aggravated the severe neck and shoulder pain I already had from working on the computer twelve to fourteen hours per day. *Was there a time in your life when you experienced physical pain, whether it was back pain, neck and shoulder pain, or headaches that just wouldn't go away?* Yes, that was my life.

After the accident, I went to see a masseuse, chiropractor, and acupuncturist—all three of them at the same time in a week. Physically, I felt better, but not great. My body still felt like there was something wrong, because I was in a state of constant aches and pain.

One day I was eating lunch at the company's kitchen, and one of the software engineers I had became good friends with came up to me and chatted. I told him I had just gotten into a really bad car accident and was having major neck and shoulder pain.

I also mentioned, "Working on the computer doesn't help with the neck and shoulder pain either."

He looked at me, paused for a second, and said with this thick Indian accent, "Awww, just go do yoga, and you'll be fine."

"Yoga?" I answered. "I'm not flexible. I can't touch my toes. Besides, yoga is for girls, right? That's not for me."

We laughed, and he repeated, "Just go do yoga."

Despite my hesitation, I decided to hear him out. I got on the Internet and found one of the many yoga centers in San Francisco. Sure enough, at my first class, there were these women in tights doing these crazy poses. *So yeah,* I thought, *yoga is probably not for me.*

A year and a half later, I went to a different company. At that time, the company was offering an introductory yoga class for free. When I started practicing yoga, I felt my body start to loosen and open up. I also felt my high stress level decrease, even though I had been working more hours than ever. Again, I ran into the same problem as practicing tai chi. The yoga sessions were more than an hour per class. Because of my busy schedule, some days I couldn't attend the yoga classes.

As I progressed through the study of tai chi and yoga, I serendipitously came across another amazing practice called qigong; the direct translation from Chinese is *energy mastery*. When I first practiced this 2,000-year-old qigong form, I immediately felt my energy flowing into the *energy rich state*. This process happened even faster than it had in any other practice, and it became the secret to uncovering my energy. It strengthened my own yoga practice, but also strengthened my internal energy as well.

Throughout my twelve years of learning, I asked my teachers and masters why I always felt better both physically and mentally after practice. I wanted to know the answer, because I wanted to reverse engineer the energy rich state, so that I could access it anytime I wanted. However, the answer I usually got from the masters was, "You don't need to know. You just need to feel."

It wasn't until I studied neuroscience that I understood how to integrate the mind with the body. After finding key secret ingredients (which I will share with you), I was able to replicate the energy rich state after each practice. It's like the law of gravity. If we move our body a certain way, we're guaranteed to feel a certain energy state.

When I applied those laws in my personal practice, my energy shot through the roof. I still worked twelve to fourteen hour days, but when I got home, I felt just as alive or vibrant as when I had gone to work. When I knew how to take care of my energy state, I became laser-sharp focused and more productive at work.

I mentioned I had worked for a high tech company. During my first quarter as a software sales account manager, I achieved more than 200 percent over my quota. In the following year, I reached more than 180 percent over my annual quota and became the number one account manager of the year.

I'm sharing this story with you not to impress you, but to let you know that I lost almost everything that I loved in my life because of my poor health. I needed to be able to pick myself back up and succeed on a massive scale.

Hopefully you don't have to experience the difficulties of what I went through in search for energy rich state. Whether you are struggling with energy or you want to bring your energy to another level, it is my sincere wish to help you have more energy in your life and share with you what is possible.

Accessing our own energy rich state is quite simple. It was eight o'clock on a Friday night as I was wrapping up work, and I was really exhausted. I didn't want to drive home immediately, because I didn't want to fall asleep behind the wheel. Instead, I did a simple fifteen-minute stress reduction technique to let go of the tension in my head and quickly recharge my mind. When I reopened my eyes after the session, one of my colleagues, Diane, who was still at work, walked up to me and said, "Wow, you're still in the office working hard? Wow, you make work seem so easy!"

"Yes, I'm still in the office, but no, it's not easy," I answered her. "I work just as hard if not harder than most people. The only difference is that I know how to charge up my energy, as I'm doing right now."

I am sure many of us can relate to working long hours and feeling exhausted. I don't know what level your energy is in your life right now.

- Maybe you are experiencing physical pain or have low energy or brain fog, and you want to be able to alleviate your pain so that you can go enjoy more of your daily life with your significant others or spouse and kids.
- Or maybe you are working in a high stress/high demand environment, and you want to alleviate stress, tensions, and headaches so that you have more concentration power and focus at work.

- Or you may want to reach the next level of your career by making sure you bring your best A game every day, so that you are even more effective and productive at work.
- Or perhaps you work in a team environment or manage a team of high achievers, and you want to have even more influence by bringing great energy and presence to lead them in high performance.

Wherever you are in life, here is my promise to you: if you go through the journey with me in this book and glean from—

- The three simple steps of my energy rich method,
- My twelve years of learning from one of the best masters whose lineage could be traced back to 2,000 years ago in ancient China,
- Combined with modern day neuroscience,

—you can experience the energy rich level on a consistent basis as well. You can feel even more alive, present, joyful, and happy!

What I'll be sharing with you took me more than a decade to learn, hone, and master. Here is the good news: you don't have to go through all of the trial and error process that I went through. I'll help you compress decades into days. I'll help you avoid pitfalls. I'll provide shortcuts to start you on the path of energy rich results. You don't need to go through six months of lying in bed with chronic stress and fatigue like I have. You don't need to travel to three different continents to learn the best energy rich methods.

When first started to share what I have learned with my close friends, they said (after my energy rich session), "When are you going to come out with DVDs? We love your methods."

Though their encouragement, I expanded my teachings at Amazon, eBay, Yahoo, HP, Cisco, VMware, and at Tony Robbins' live seminars. My clients loved it. They said, "We've never experienced anything like this before. We feel energetic all day, and we didn't even need to drink coffee. We love your classes."

And this is why I am excited to share with you this book. If you allow me to guide you in this journey, I'm going to share with you the most powerful energy rich methods I have developed. I believe you're going to love the process, and it is my sincere wish that I will help you save time and shorten the learning curve.

Are you intrigued with what is really possible for your life now? If you were to imagine where your energy is today and where you really want to be, would your life be even more successful? How would your love life be—when you came back home full of energy and presence with your spouse and kids? What would life be like if you experienced even more joy, happiness, and excitement—with the energy rich you can create at your fingertips?

Hey isn't this true?

"If you don't have energy, you're not going to be able to focus at work, much less be productive."

"If you don't have energy, you're not going to influence anybody because no one wants to hangout with negative people."

"If you don't have energy, you can't do a great job raising your kids because they'll run all over you."

I promise you that if you master your energy, not only will you be even more productive at work, but you will see a difference in the other parts of your life that matter even more because **"Energy is LIFE!"**

Ready to get started?

I also want to take a moment to honor you for reading this far, because you are the top 10 percent of the population who wants to take their lives to the next level. Yes, that's correct! Statistic shows that less than 10 percent of people who buy a nonfiction book read past the first chapter. Isn't that crazy? So here is your first energy rich exercise – Raise your right hand, palm facing up. Reach up your right arm. Bend your elbow and pat yourself on the back!

I have written this book to help you simply build massive momentum into your life—while also offering you enough depth to master your energy rich level. This will give you even more focus and productivity—and the ability to be more influential to your team.

I put together very simple methods based on four powerful sections:

Secret Energy Hack Section I – Jump Start Your Own Energy Naturally

Secret Energy Hack Section II – What Drains Our Life Energy?

Secret Energy Hack Section III – Manage Your Energy for Life

Secret Energy Hack Section IV – The Joy of Pure Energy

I offer an invitation to you now and challenge you to take this journey with me through all of the sections. I promise you that when you are living the energy rich life, it will spill over into every aspect of your life. You will reap the rewards when you implement what learn in this book.

How do you get your energy for the next month, next year, and decades to come? I'm going to show you how to *master and reach your own energy rich level.*

That is what this book is really about. Let's turn the page, and let me give you a brief overview of what it will take to master your energy rich level for life.

Ready to jump-start your own energy rich level? **Go to www.AllanTing.com/IEMBookBonuses** to claim your free bonuses. You will get an eight minutes instant stress relief audio meditation MP3 and a fifteen minutes body balance exercise video.

Introduction

"Every important mistake I've made in my life,
I've made because I was too tired."

— Bill Clinton

Let me ask you this. Have you ever worked with a boss or manager—or someone on your team—who was grumpy and miserable? This person was always so serious, and you felt like he was a ticking time bomb waiting to go off? On certain days, maybe you've had coworkers spreading instant messages around the office saying, "John is really *agro* today, so stay away from him like the plague."

Then we walk as fast as we can past John's office with a stack of paper in our hands, pretending to be reading something really important, just to avoid striking up a conversation with "the bad mood boss." What's worse is we feel like we can't approach management with questions or advice about work, because we don't want to be the spark that sets off the already short fuse. So instead, we push off the question until the boss is in a better mood, which often delays key critical business decisions.

Think of the Dwight Schrute character in the TV series, *The Office,* and how everyone tries to avoid him. Doesn't Dwight bring everyone's mood and energy down with his sadistic demeanor?

Yes, absolutely! When we have a poor energy level, we affect the people around us and bring down their energy, too.

Tiredness results in bad energy. Bad energy results in negative thoughts. Negative thoughts result in bad moods. Bad moods affect the people around them; no one can lead a high performing team when the influencer is miserable and angry all the time.

On the flip side, when we are happy and flowing in the energy rich zone, don't we bring that good mood to our workplace, clients, and family? And when we feel alive, don't the people around us respond back with good energy? Sure, they do!

One thing for sure is that we can't influence anyone if we are in a bad mood. No one wants to work with a tyrant boss.

That is why it is so important to learn how to manage our own energy.

Have you heard of a very successful online shoe company called Zappos? How does Zappos thrive and beat out many of their retail competitors? How does Zappos have so many raving fans, when their shoe prices aren't the lowest in the industry? One of their core beliefs is to build a positive team and family spirit. This is how they attract very talented people to work for them. Who wouldn't want to hang out with positive people who are fun, passionate, and energy rich?

So how do we have more focus, be more productive, and be a person of influence on our teams?

To be a high performer, we need to build strong fundamentals— the right mindset and body—to help us to be even more successful. Building the right fundamentals will only help us amplify more energy, instill a good mood, and let us enjoy the quality of an extraordinary life.

One fall afternoon in 2001, I went on a run in San Francisco's Golden Gate Park, while holding a portable CD player and listening to Tony Robbins as he was talking about building an extraordinary life—life on our terms. As I got closer to the Polo Field and began smelling the freshly cut grass, Tony started to tell a story about when he took his kids to watch Cirque du Soleil in his hometown of Del Mar, California. As Tony and his family were getting ready to sit down and enjoy the show in the VIP section, he noticed that there were three empty premium seats missing and he thought, "Wow, someone is going to miss out on an amazing show."

Just then, "...a giant man, walking with the help of a cane and two assistants, came down the stairs. He must have weighed at least 400 pounds." When the overly obese man sat down, he took three of those empty seats and "...was wheezing and sweating from the short walk to the front row." As he sat down, his overweight body parts rolled out of his seat and crushed Tony's daughter who sat right next to him! Tony overheard someone behind him saying that "...he was the richest man in Canada."

Tony felt so badly for the person. It turned out that he was one of the billionaires in Canada, but he had put so much of his attention in making money that he neglected his physical health. "And by failing to master more than one aspect of his life, he couldn't enjoy what he had, not even a simple, magical evening at the theater."

But here is the problem. Tell me this: when you went through school, did your education lead you to believe that you needed to get good grades? Because getting good grades meant that you had a greater chance at getting into a great college, right? And getting into a great college meant that you had a greater chance to get a great job after you get out. Then you would climb the corporate ladder, and when you attained the VP title and made a six figure or higher income, then you would be somebody, right?

Isn't it true that in our culture, success is defined by how much money we have and what our status is? *The more money or power you have, the more successful you are,* so we believe.

Our success is rarely or never measured by health and happiness.

You and I both know that if we don't take time to care for our health, money doesn't matter. We can try to make more money, but something feels like it's missing and life doesn't feel fulfilled. The old metaphor, "the richest man in the graveyard," comes into play when we don't have the health, the vitality, or the energy.

But often, don't we put health as the least of our priorities? It's all about perspective when we hear that someone we love got cancer and has three more months to live. We pause, take a step back, and re-evaluate what is important in our lives, don't we? It's that moment when we realize that perhaps we should put health first.

If we look at recent research and news, however, we see that material or career success does not necessarily buy us health and joy—and in fact can deter from it. *Business Insider* published an article on May 8, 2013, titled, "Burnout Is Such a Huge Problem," suggesting that the lifestyle of a typical CEO is almost perfectly designed to burn out those people. A Harvard Medical School study cited in the article found that about 96 percent of senior management felt somewhat burnt out, and one-third of them described their burnout as extreme.

Do you know of someone who is successful, by society's definition at least—perhaps with the million-dollar yacht, the fancy house, and all of the best wines he can drink? Sure, we all do. They often are addicted to drugs, alcohol, or food—even though they are at the top. They are still miserable, aren't they?

I was talking to a good friend of mine who coaches America's top executives. She said that one of her clients is the CEO of a large, publicly traded pet store chain. His problem isn't in meeting the shareholders' expectations. Rather, he most fears having a heart attack and not being able to walk his daughter down the aisle at her wedding.

Oh by the way, speaking of money and happiness, Gallup surveyed 450,000 Americans to find out if there is a correlation between happiness and money. The theory is, "If we made more money, the happier we would be." While it's true that we need money to cover our basic necessities like food, water, shelter, guess what income level the study found that happiness flat-lined—meaning that happiness levels didn't increase after making above this level of income?

Is it the million dollars that we're after? Would we be happier if we made $10 million—and then we'd be much, much happier?

The research showed that after $75,000, people weren't get much happier. Anything after that, people just bought more things, and they weren't happier.

Do you remember the actor Philip Seymour Hoffman from the movie, *Hunger Games?* Philip had so many things going for him. He was a very talented actor who won an Oscar and received many other nominations, but his success did not equate to health. On February 2, 2014, he was found dead in his New York apartment with a syringe in his left arm. At age forty-six, he had overdosed from drugs. He had everything going for him—fame and money—but why did he still die? *It's because he failed to take good care of his mind and his body.*

Why am I giving so many examples of why health is important? Most of us intellectually understand the importance of health as a concept, but not many of us apply what we have learned. Or we might eat healthy food and work out on a regular basis, but how often do we pay close attention to our emotional health?

Most Americans spend more time planning a vacation than paying close attention to their health and what they eat. One of the first things we need to do if we want to be truly successful at life is to get our health back to normal. *When we're healthy, we are full of energy—and everything is possible in this state.*

So whether you want even more success having more focus, being more productive, or being able to influence your team, you need to have rich energy to take care of your mind and body first. When you have the fundamentals down, that's when you can repeat success over and over.

You may be asking, *"How do I live in the energy rich state on a consistent basis?"*

Let's go over a few questions to benchmark your energy level day in and day out. If I knocked on your door and came to live with you for a month, where would your energy level be on a regular basis? By the way, be as honest as you can, so that you know how to level up! Let me ask you:

- **Do you get short bursts of energy and then easily get tired?**
- **Are you exhausted and barely holding your head above water?**
- **Do you just want to lie in bed and do nothing?**

Let's first define the four states of energy so that we know where we are so that we know where we are and how to change our state.

The Energy State Quadrant

Quadrant 1	Quadrant 2
Energy Rich Energy Lasting	Energy Rich Energy Non-Lastiing
Quadrant 3	Quadrant 4
Energy Poor Exhaustion	Energy Poor Lethargic

Quadrant 1: Energy Rich, Energy Lasting State

Living in the energy rich and energy rich state, we experience massive momentum in our lives. We feel unstoppable, like we are on a mission. We feel present, alive, joyful, happy, and free. We jump out of our beds every morning and can't wait to get our days started. We love what we do at work, even if we don't get paid. We're in great health, our energy is rich and abundant, and our diet is excellent. Our relationships are great, and we love life. We live a very passionate life, and we see problems as challenges. We continue to improve ourselves, grow every day, and contribute back into society. We live in this energy rich, energy abundant quadrant day in and day out for decades.

Quadrant 2: Energy Rich, Energy Non-Lasting State

Many of you probably have experienced the energy rich state and felt absolutely alive at some point in your lives—such as when you accomplished something great that you never thought you could do. Perhaps it was overcoming the fear of heights when you skydived for the first time. Or perhaps it was the feeling of accomplishment while crossing the finish line at your first marathon. It could also have been the feeling of victory when your favorite baseball team won the World's Series. Or it could have been the heart falling feeling when you fell in love and kissed your partner for the first time. It's that exuberating feeling that life is grand. You feel on top of the world, and that nothing will stop you.

What was life like when you experienced the energy rich state? Were you much happier? When you ran into any challenges—whether they were work or relationship related—you stood up to those challenges better, didn't you?

Then what happened? Did the momentum keep going, or did the energy rich state slowly taper off and even start to decline?

Most of us have experienced the energy rich state; but at some point, the energy tapered off and gradually lowered back into the energy poor state. In other words, the energy rich state is not sustainable. We go back to the status quo. Then, when someone asks you, "How is it going?" you say, "Meh, it's alright" or, "It's going."

There are two main reasons why we have the tendency to drop back into the status quo.

The first reason is peer pressure from those we hang around with. Have you ever been vibrant, happy, and full of energy—and then you overheard someone saying about you, "Why is she so damn happy? What drug is she on?" Even though maybe you were at an energy state of 9 (out of 10), you quickly drop your enthusiastic energy state down to a 5 or 6 so that you don't upset others.

As a high performer, we can't let other people dictate our energy rich state, because we all deserve to live in the energy rich state. If anything, we should strive to have people coming up to us and asking, "How do you do it? How do you feel so alive?"

The second reason is that we experience the energy rich state and then become complacent. We forget that experiencing the energy rich state requires consistent practice. We can't go to the gym one time and expect to be fit for the rest of our lives. Similarly, in experiencing the energy rich and energy rich state, we also need to continually build those emotional and physical muscles.

What if you could experience this energy rich state on a consistent basis? How would it feel to live in that powerful state? Pretty awesome, huh? The truth is, we can live in the energy rich state consistently if we know the right strategy.

In this book, you'll learn a 2,000-year-old, ancient secret Chinese practice that will help you get to the energy rich state. This is a practice that Oprah and Dr. Oz highly recommend as well.

Quadrant 3: Energy Poor, Exhaustion State

I'm sure most of us have experienced exhaustion and burnout at some times in our lives. For some of us, we live on a daily basis barely keeping our heads above water. I was invited to talk on "ABC Newsroom" recently about how to experience more rich energy in our lives. As I was on the set getting miked up for sound, the news anchor said to me, "Do you have any advice for exhaustion? I can't sleep at night, and I have a hard time getting up in the morning."

I asked her how long she had been experiencing this, and she said, "It's been so long that I can't remember."

I said to her, "You need to be alive and present on TV, so having energy is really important at your job, isn't it?"

She perked up her ears, nodded her head and said, "Yes. Having energy is crucial at my line of work. So how can I get more energy naturally?" she asked.

"I will demo the quick pick-me-up, energy exercise during our interview, and you tell me if you feel more alive afterwards," I smiled.

Afterwards, she couldn't thank me enough for helping her perform at her job. She felt the most alive she had in recent months. But first, I had to show her how to plug the energy draining holes first.

Quadrant 4: Energy Poor, Lethargic State

This state is probably the easiest from which to level up to quadrant 1 and 2 of the energy rich state and because it is the easiest, I'm only going to address it in this section of the book. However it does require one thing: we need to get our butts off the couch and go exercise.

Have you ever been lying on the couch watching *Oprah* while eating a tub of Häagen-Dazs, vanilla ice cream? I mean, it's one of those days when you just want to lie there and sing to the tune of Bruno Mars' "The Lazy Song": "Today I don't feel like doing anything, I just wanna lay in my bed, Don't feel like picking up my phone, So leave a message at the tone, 'Cause today I swear I'm not doing anything."

I know this scenario only because I have been there. I'm only teasing you because I care!

The states of feeling lazy or lethargic are different than that of exhaustion. Exhaustion means you worked your butt off and didn't get enough rest. Lethargy suggests a lack of motivation.

This is when you need to stay away from your sofa, even when it's calling your name, "Mary, come sit and relax with me. Come sit for just five minutes."

Don't cave in to sitting on the couch. Just don't do it! Stay away from it, and go for a walk or run or to the gym. Remember the object in motion stays in motion. The reverse is also true, when our butts are glued to the couch!

Have you ever regretted working out afterwards? Most likely not! That's why getting to the gym is half the battle. Go take a power or flow yoga class. You'll be glad you did, and you can pat yourself on the back afterwards.

What Not to Do

Before we cover how to get the most out of this book, I want to talk about *what not to* do as you read it. If you want more energy in your life, you've got to keep an eye the following.

The first thing to focus on is your diet. If you eat like crap—meaning if you eat junk food all of the time—this book is not going to help you, point blank. If you eat mostly pizza, hamburgers, and fried chicken—or if you eat only meat or a non-plant based type of diet—I'm sorry, but this book is not going to get you more energy. Don't get me wrong, I do enjoy life and have a good double double In-N-Out burger once in a blue moon—but it's not my main diet. If you clean up your diet and apply the rest of what I introduce in this book, your energy is going to skyrocket. It's going to boom! It's going to burst into space.

The second thing to focus on is sleep. As a high performance coach, I was working with a young and passionate college professor recently, and he wanted my help to get more productive at work. He said, "You know, I love my work—teaching college biology—

but I feel like I'm not being productive enough. Sometimes, in fact, I feel flat out lazy, and I don't want to do anything."

I asked him the same question I had asked the news anchor, "How many hours do you sleep a night?"

He said, "I force myself to sleep three to five hours per day."

I asked him, "How is sleeping three to five hours per day working out for you?"

He responded, "Well, to be honest with you, it's not really working at all."

"When you are tired and groggy and lecturing, and you're teaching your students—how effective is that?" I waited for his answer.

He paused. "Yeah, you're right Allan. It's not really effective at all."

"And how well are you serving your students as their professor?"

He sighed. "I am not."

It is a false belief that we can get ahead by sleeping less, because when we do, we are even more tired and less productive. In the old world, people thought, *"Hey, I only need to sleep four to five hours a day, so that I can be more productive."* Research has proven that this strategy backfires. Bill Clinton used to sleep only five hours a night, and he admitted that the important mistakes he made were because of lack of sleep. One of the most extensive studies done on sleep deprivation was conducted in the military during the first Iraqi war and also post war with America's elite forces—the Navy Seals and Army Rangers. The military found that the less soldiers slept, the more their stress levels increased. Most of all, their key critical decision-making skills dropped exponentially with lack of sleep and caused catastrophic events.

Colonel Gregory Belenky, director of the Division of Neuroscience for the US Army Medical Corps, case studied one of the well-documented friendly fire incidents during the first Gulf

War, wherein a group of M2 Bradley tanks fired on each other. The soldiers had been awake for forty-eight hours during the assault. They mistook the friendly tanks for enemies. Even though the tankers were able to operate simple tasks such as driving the tanks, the study concluded that soldiers had a much harder time deciphering complicated tasks with little sleep.

"When time runs out and the person has not been able to reach an accurate decision, the person is forced to guess" (Belenky, Marcy, and Martin).

If the person is a part of a complicated network of systems and makes a fatal mistake, such as the tank commander who ordered the gunner to fire at the friendlies, disaster occurs and the system falls apart.

To further prove that sleep deprivation causes problems, the army also studied soldiers' brains after twenty-four hours of no sleep using PET scans. The images showed a significant decrease in the parts of the brain that are responsible for attention, planning, and anticipation, which explained the brain fog from the friendly-fire case study.

Fortunately, most of us live in a non-combatant zone and probably never experience the amount of stress from life-threatening situations and lack of sleep as soldiers would. However, like the military, corporations also have a chain of command that typically includes a board of directors, CEO, CFO, CTO, VPs, and managers. Each corporation is a network of complicated processes. If a financial controller overlooks the financial statement because he is burnt-out and didn't get enough sleep, and the CFO signs off on the 10-K annual report filed to the SEC, the CFO could be subjected to fines, imprisonment, or both due to non-Sarbanes Oxley compliancy.

Mistakes happen, because we're human. I recall how frantic the finance departments became at the end of a quarter when

I worked at well-known high tech companies. As an account manager, I would stay until 1:30 a.m. to make sure the accounting department accepted all of my purchase orders. They burned the big jug of midnight oil, staying up all night to finish booking all of the transactions. That was the standard operation every quarter.

Want to guess how many hours the military recommends our soldiers sleep if at all possible? You got it. It's eight hours.

We'll talk more about neuroplasticity and how our brain functions later in the book, so that we can develop our own mental capacity to focus and achieve our goals. For the time being, you want be on top of your game, don't you? You want to have more confidence, creativity, and even better decision making processes and leadership skills, yes? Then let's turn off your lights and get some good night rest, people!

The third thing to pay attention to is your alcohol consumption. There is this miscommunication from doctors: "Hey, if you drink red wine, it's great for your heart." But the pulmonary doctors don't talk to the neuro doctors. Yes, the wine is great for your heart, and it keeps your blood moving. However, from a neuroscience perspective, that formaldehyde is killing your brain cells. The NIH Institute on Alcohol Abuse and Alcoholism reports, " Long-term heavy drinking may lead to shrinking of the brain and deficiencies in the fibers (white matter) that carry information between brain cells (gray matter)."

So it might be good for your heart, but what good is a heart if your brain cells are dying? Drink in moderation, or try not to drink at all.

The fourth thing is if you do drugs, such as narcotics, I'm sorry, I can't help you. You may have seen the movie, *Dallas Buyers Club*. It's about Matthew McConaughey's character going through his own journey. He was diagnosed with AIDS, but the reason he stayed alive for another nine or ten years is because he lived a very healthy lifestyle. He started eating a plant based, vegetable diet. He stopped drinking alcohol, and his life turned around. He communicated to his friend that the most important thing was to stay alive, and that they should stop doing drugs and eat better food.

The fifth thing you have to know is how to manage your stress level. A lot of people consider themselves healthy. They say, "I don't eat junk food," but there are emotional toxins and stress that affect you similarly to the things you eat. There are lots of combinations and pieces of the puzzle.

How to Get the Most Out of This Book?

We talked about what not to do, so let's talk about how to help you get the most out of this book. Darren Hardy, author of the *NY Times* bestseller *Compound Effect,* said, "What is easy to do is also easy not to do." My methodology is based on things that are very simple *to do.*

If you look at high achievers, what distinguish them from others are the things they do as fundamental. The people are not any different in their makeup. They don't have superpowers. However, they do certain things over and over again. These actions are simple, but because the achievers do them, they have consistency—and health. They have discipline and are able to achieve more. Remember we discussed that having the right fundamentals will help you amplify your energy and happiness? Why not model the people who are successful? Why reinvent the wheel? When they wake up in the morning, there are specific things that the most successful achievers do before breakfast. They spend some time by themselves, for example. Tony Robbins calls it "five minutes of thrive, fifteen minutes of fulfillment, or an hour of power." Some of us don't have that hour, because we have kids, we have to drop them off at school, we have to do a whole bunch of other things. We have obligations. I get that. That's why I've broken out the exercises in this book into sections of five minutes, fifteen minutes, and a half hour.

Ideally, you will want to do my sequences for a half hour in the morning and then five minutes throughout the day. Then, in the afternoon when you're stressed, you can do my fifteen minute stress reliever. One of my students, Betty, told me that just doing my fifteen minute sections lowers her blood pressure by ten points.

Knowledge itself is not power. Knowledge on its own is only a concept with potential value. The execution of knowledge is where your power lies. So in simple terms, knowing is not enough, like Bruce Lee said. You have to turn that into action.

And that's part of the learning curve as well, because when we learn, we go through three types of mastery.

1. **The first step is called intellectual mastery.** We know it by heart, but if we don't do it, what's the point? It's useless, right?
2. **The second step is to bring intellectual mastery and emotional mastery into the picture.** We feel it, we understand it needs to be done, we understand the reason why. But if we still don't do it—we don't take action—it's still not going to get us anywhere.
3. **That's why we need the third part, called *physical mastery.*** Until we start to get physical with it and actually take action—moving our body—we're just holding all the knowledge without letting it transform us.

I have written this book to help you get 80 percent of the results with 20 percent of the effort. I am a true believer of the KISS model, Keep it Simple and Sweet, which means that I am giving simple and practical, bite-sized information and exercises. Everything I talk about and teach in this book is practical.

I strongly invite you to read this book, and at the same time, do the exercises. Besides the exercises, there will be homework. I highly encourage you to engage in action with the activities, because you're going to get the most out of your experience if you do. You've already invested your time and money in reading my book. So why not get the most from it, right?

Don't forget to get your free bonuses that come with this book. **Go to www.AllanTing.com/IEMBookBonuses to claim your free bonus.** You get an eight minutes instant stress relief audio meditation MP3 and a fifteen minutes body balance exercise video.

Best of Both Worlds –
Ancient Practice Meets Modern Science

So how did I hone my expertise in all of this? As I mentioned, in 2001, I suffered from chronic stress and fatigue syndrome. I didn't want to stay in bed for the rest of my life, so I started learning Eastern energy practices and Eastern medicine. I started learning yoga, Eastern arts, tai chi, and qigong; but I felt like there was still something missing. It wasn't until I started studying neuro-linguistic programming (NLP) and neuroscience that I felt a huge shift. So, when I combined everything—yoga, the mindfulness practice, the Zen meditation that Steve Jobs also practiced, and qigong and tai chi with NLP with neuroscience—I was able to find the answer.

For the longest time, I would finish a yoga class, and an hour or an hour and a half later, and I would feel great. I'd ask my teachers, "Why do I feel great?" and nobody could answer me. They might try to discuss it from a philosophical perspective, but nobody could explain it to me from a scientific perspective.

It wasn't until started studying neuroscience that I realized the reasons why I felt better. Let me ask you, if you were to picture a depressed person who was sitting down, what would his body posture look like? Would he be a) sitting tall, or b) slouched forward?

You'll say that this person's head would probably be bopping down a little bit low, and his shoulders would probably be hunched. Right? That is just how we are hard wired. It's like the laws of gravity. It doesn't matter who in the world you are observing or who you are—whether you're a man or a woman, if you grew up in America, if you grew up in France, if you grew up in South Africa—we're all built that way. And once you understand that, we can start unlocking our potentials. These are the GPS to our mind and body.

When we buy a new laptop, it comes with a manual. When we were born, no one gave us a manual on how our brain works. Our brain is this very complicated computer system, which requires specific care to function optimally. But once you understand the fundamentals, you can make a huge shift in your life to fine tune how you operate—and maximize what you are able to achieve by knowing how to move our body.

What new distinctions about energy have you learned so far? Are you convinced that you should get at least 7-9 hours of sleep a day?

Keep up the good work! We're about to roll up our sleeves and get going in the next chapter but before that, would you do me a small favor? Do you know a friend that might be able to benefit from the book? If so, I love to have you share this book link **www.AllanTing.com/IEMBook** to your friend. Thanks in advance.

Jump Start Your Own Energy Naturally – POW

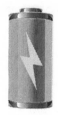

<u>P</u>osture
<u>O</u>xygen
<u>W</u>ater

Secret Energy Hack Section I Overview

"Nothing tastes as good as absolute health and energy."
— Tony Robbins

I met Jack Canfield through an expert association a few years ago. One of the characteristics about Jack that I respect is that he is a down-to-earth person who practices kindness and patience, even though he has sold more than five hundred million copies of *Chicken Soup for the Soul* worldwide. He hasn't let success go to his head.

It was about eight-thirty p.m., and we were wrapping up from a very long day at the conference. Jack was on his way back to his hotel room, when a mob of more than one hundred people engulfed him. I'm pretty sure Jack had had a long day too. He had flown in to give a standing ovation speech. He hadn't had dinner yet. He was most likely tired and wanting to go back to his hotel room. Instead, Jack stood there and talked to each one of us individually for at least five minutes. The security guard came over and wanted to escort Jack away from the long line of people, but Jack stood his ground and told the security guard that he was okay with the crowd.

And here is the lesson I learned from Jack that day that I want to share with you: *if we are okay with ourselves—meaning if we are overflowing with energy—we are able to serve and connect more with others.* It's like what flight attendants do when they conduct a safety briefing before take-off. When you're on an airplane and the masks drop, what do they tell you to do? Should you put the mask on other people first? No, you put it on yourself first—*before* helping your children...and *then* your husband! That was a joke one of the flight attendants cracked when I was on Southwest Airlines.

See, we have to get our own energy up. We have to feel more alive *first*. High performers don't wait for others to start. We get going first, don't we? Once we have the energy, we can better serve other people.

Now, imagine if Jack had been angry or exhausted; he might have been irritated. If he had been irritated, would he have stood there and talked to all of us? Most likely, he would have needed to retreat back to his room, or at least would not have been as engaged with his fans. Instead, Jack was very present, and was there to talk to and serve every single one of us.

When we are taking care of ourselves and are full of energy, whether it's happiness, love, or gratitude, we're able to contribute more to our families and the people around us. Similarly, when we love our self, our love overflows, and everyone around us will feel it too.

We do no good for anybody if we're tired all the time, so we have to know how to take care of ourselves by generating our own energy naturally.

Generating your own energy isn't as hard as you think. You don't need to rely on coffee. We all can generate our own energy naturally.

Two months ago, I did something crazy. Given the time constraint, I had to attend two live seminars back to back and travel around the county for thirteen days with an average of three hours of sleep per night. I did it without any caffeine or energy drinks.

Admittedly, it was not the brightest idea. Going into it, it almost felt like a suicide mission, but as a high performer, don't we love to take on challenges?

My journey started with traveling to the KTLA Fox 5 lot in Los Angeles for four days to kick-start my national media tour. I had an intense two days of media training followed by two more days of intense pitching to TV news producers across the country about my book.

A good friend of mine recommended that I check out AirBnB, since he had great luck staying at luxurious houses for fractions of the full prices. I found a plush house 1.5 miles from the KTLA station for 50 bucks a night. I scored—or at least I thought I did. It turned out that it was four bunk beds in a tiny 350-square-foot space, and my two other roommates snored all through the night. I had full digital surround sound, as if I were in an Imax Theater.

On the second night, the owner of the house approached me and said, "Oh by the way, I forgot to tell you. My partner recently passed, so we're throwing a goodbye party for him."

I said to her, "I am a pretty concerned, because tomorrow is a very important day. I need all of my energy to pitch in front of TV news producers. I really need to get a good night's rest."

She affirmed me with, "Well, the party shouldn't pass 1 a.m., so that means you should be able to get some rest."

I finally got back home at 11:30 p.m. that night after an exhausting day of intense media training, and guess what I walked into? Beats of loud hip-hop music—and people chatting up a storm, laughing, having a good time, and smoking varieties of dry leaves.

I walked past a cloud of weed dust to climb up to my second level bunk bed, put on my Bose noise cancelling headset, curled up in bed, and went to sleep. Well, kind of. I woke at 3:30 a.m. to the sound of girls crying and inhaling secondhand cigarette smoke. I couldn't get back to sleep thinking about my pitches to the news producers in a few short hours.

Pitching to new producers is like pitching in front of Kevin Harrington on the TV show, Shark Tank. You bring your highest energy and smiling-until-my-cheeks-hurt face, conveying why the producers should book you on their show. There were ten of us, and we had three minutes each to pitch to twelve producers across the country. If the producers liked us, we'd be booked on their news stations. It was so stressful that some participants broke down and froze during the middle of their pitches.

Even though I was operating on a few hours of sleep and no coffee, I was able to successfully pitch to the producers. Out of the eleven producers there, I got ten bookings from ABC, NBC, CBS, Fox, and CW News across the country all by doing very simple and effective energy boosting exercises.

What happened during the next nine days when I was extremely sleep deprived and had to attend my seminar trip—including coaching two seminar attendees who wanted to commit suicide? (Yes, they had experienced very traumatic events in their lives.) I really had to step up my energy level to serve them. I will share details with you later, but first, let me help you springboard your energy into Quadrant 2–Energy Rich, Energy Not Lasting.

You might be wondering why I'm not teaching you Quadrant 1–Energy Rich, Energy Lasting yet, and there is a reason why. It's because you need to know how to boost your energy first as a foundation before moving on to the advanced energy method. Be patient "grasshoppa." I promise I'll show you the way.

Quadrant 1 Energy Rich Energy Lasting	Quadrant 2 Energy Rich Energy Non-Lasting
Quadrant 3 Energy Poor Exhaustion	Quadrant 4 Energy Poor Lethargic

In the rest of this section, I'm going to share three simple and very powerful ways to boost your energy based on my Posture, Oxygen, and Water (POW) Method. During the short period of thirteen days of my trip, I focused on these three things to boost my energy whenever I felt my energy level take a drive, and I am going to detail how you can, too!

I am going to point out many practical and common sense frameworks throughout this book to help boost and maintain your energy. You might be saying, "Yeah, posture, oxygen, and water are common sense. I don't need to buy a book about it." But common sense is not always common practice, is it?

Why don't we read and find out just what science says about POW—Posture, Oxygen, Water?

CHAPTER 1

First Energy Booster: Watch Your Posture

"Honey, don't slouch!"

— Your mother

The first key cornerstone of mastering your energy is to pay very close attention to your posture, because how we stand affects our energy, our body's biochemistry, our hormones, and how we feel about ourselves.

We know that successful, high performers are more energetic, more dominant, more optimistic, and more apt to take risks—because they are more confident. If I were to ask you what a high performer's body posture looks like, what would you say?

- Would her posture be more open?
- Would she be standing tall?
- Would her shoulders be back and her chin up?

My bet is that you'll say, "All of the above!"

Recently, ABC, NBC, and Fox News invented me on their news segments to talk about one of the worst mistakes to avoid if we want to have more energy in our lives. The first thing I asked the TV reporter was, "What does our posture look like when we are checking our stock quotes, texting our spouse, or Facebooking on our iPhones?"

The anchors laughed and said, "Um…We are slouching and leaning forward!"

I said, "Yes, and this posture is so bad for our energy."

When we don't pay attention to our poor posture—when we're typing away on our iPhones, iPad, or laptops, or reading on our Kindle—we are conditioning our bodies to have low energy. Most people aren't even aware of their own bad posture. You know that concave dinosaur pose you take when staring at a computer screen? The one where your hips pivot forward, your back is rounded out, and your neck is straining forward at an awkward 15-degree angle while you knock out "just one more email" at your computer?

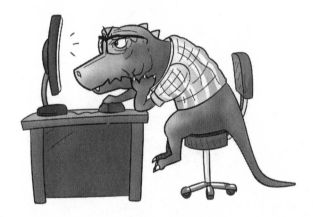

I bet many of you are doing the same pose right now! Freeze! Don't move, and check your own posture! You probably sat up a bit taller, didn't you? You're busted!

We have a term for that here in the Silicon Valley. We call it *Silicon Valley Syndrome*. Is this familiar? Yes, I had it too!

When we compress our spines, we also compress thousands of nervous endings in our spinal column and all of our internal organs as well. Not to mention that bad posture affects our mood and confidence, as Harvard studies have shown.

That's why it's so important that you watch your posture. When you have the awareness and consistently keep great posture, your body will feel more open and your energy floodgate will open. There is a reason why our moms always nagged us: "Don't slouch." Let's dive deeply into how poor posture affects our lives and what Harvard social psychologist, Amy Cuddy, and her colleagues report from their research.

In Cuddy's June 2012 TED Talk, "Your Body Language Shapes Who You Are," she revealed her research about how posture affects our everyday lives. She asked participants to spit into vials to collect their saliva samples and then had them adopt different postures of high power and low power. One test group held a high-power posture and the other test group held a low-power posture for two minutes. Then the researchers gave them an opportunity to gamble and recollected their saliva to see if there was any biochemical change.

Biochemically, those with confident postures had a rise in testosterone, or the "dominance hormone," and lower cortisol, or the "stress hormone" (a 20 percent increase in testosterone level and a 25 percent decrease in cortisol). Those who slouched had a decrease in testosterone and increase in cortisol (10 percent decrease in testosterone and 15 percent increase in cortisol).

It's very important to note that the participants in the Harvard study only held either the high-power posture or low-power posture for two minutes! In just two minutes, researchers saw a radical change in their bodies' biochemistry (Cuddy, Wilmuth, and Carney).

Imagine if we held a low-power posture day in and day out. How would that condition our energy, confidence, mood, and lives? The correlation is common sense, but not common practice, right?

In a moment here, I will demonstrate how to open up your body to allow your energy to start to follow—with proper breathing, which leads to point number two.

CHAPTER 2

Second Energy Booster: Oxygenate Your Body

"There is no single more powerful—or more simple—daily practice to further your health and well being than breathwork."

— Andrew Weil, MD

Improper breathing is a common cause of ill health. If I had to limit my advice on healthier living to just one tip, it would be simply to learn how to breathe correctly.

The second key cornerstone to health and vitality is oxygen. Within the topic of oxygen, there are two sub-areas that I want to cover:

1. The first is how decreased oxygen impacts our cells, and
2. Second, how breathing can help us regulate our nervous system and control the way we feel.

First, we all know that if we don't get oxygen, we will die, because our brain cells that govern the functions of our entire bodies would die. But most of us don't know how lower oxygen affects our cells.

What if I were to tell you that cells could live forever under the right conditions? That is exactly what Dr. Alexis Carrel, a two-time Nobel Prize winner, proved to the world. He was able to extract cells from a chicken and keep them alive on petri dishes twenty-seven years later. The experiment went so well that the cells outlived Dr. Carrel, proving his theory that "cells will live forever" under the right environment—without toxins and given their basic needs, such as oxygen. Dr. Carrel was able to keep cells alive. But what things would have destroyed the living cells? All that the scientists needed to do was to eliminate oxygen in the petri dishes, interrupt the electrical field of the cells, or physically tear the cell linings. If they did any of those three, the cells would die.

Now that we have discussed how oxygen affects our cells, second, let's talk about how breathing affects our nervous systems. Most people are not aware of their breath, because their bodies govern their inhalation and exhalation automatically. But most people also don't understand the *power* of their breath—and why it is important to breathe consciously and consistently.

Do you breathe consciously and purposely? I know I don't do it very often. Most of us don't. If you want to have more energy in your life, you've got to do what I call *conscious breathing*—because if you are like most people, so much of your life is on autopilot.

Let's do a quick exercise. I'd like you to think about your commute to work five days ago. Do you remember everyone you encountered on your way to work? Do you remember all the different colors of the cars you saw? Heck, how about the clothes you were wearing?

For most of us, we just know that we left the house and got to work. Most of everything in between we don't remember, because our lives are on automatic pilot. That is a picture of our stressful, modern day in the life—because we have bigger fish to fry at work.

If you want more vital energy in your life, you need to learn how to harness your breath. This is not a new phenomenon. We simply forget the power of our breath.

Many ancient languages talk about breath in association with mind, body, and spirit. *Aloha*—which we know as "hello" in Hawaiian—comes from two words: *alo*, meaning the center of the universe, and *ha*, the breath. Another example is the word "inspiration," which comes from the ancient Latin word root *spiritus*, meaning spirit or breath. The Chinese call it "qi," which means "life-force energy" or "breath of heaven."

A few years ago, I traveled with a few colleagues on a business trip. While sitting at San Francisco International Airport waiting to board our plane, I pulled out a book from my laptop bag and started to read. My colleague who was sitting across from me glanced at my book and said, "Allan, what are you reading over there? A book titled *A Life Worth Breathing*? Are you an idiot? Don't you know how to breathe?"

I laughed, shook my head and smiled.

In our society and schools, we were never taught how to manage stress, tension, anxiety, and fear. I don't remember any classes offered in my high school or college about stress reduction. Adolescence is when we go through the most amount of change, both physically and mentally, and stress in our lives.

The only time people learn about how to manage stress is during pregnancy—and what is the one important key the classes teach? It is breathing. If women go through that much pain during pregnancy, and they've been taught to breathe, maybe we should adopt breathing into our own stressful lives. Because when we become aware with our breathing, we can manage our emotions and stress level.

Let's take a close look at breathing. If I were to ask you to picture someone who is stressed out and under tremendous pressure from work, how would he breathe? Would he breathe fully and open—or shallow and closed?

Yes, he is breathing shallow and closed. This is common sense, because we have experienced it ourselves, and we have seen it in other people, but not common knowledge. Through breathing, we can change how we feel. We can change our state from one of stress to one that is calm and relaxed in a matter of seconds.

We need to know how to modulate our breath. But first we need to be aware of our breath.

Our breath is the connector of our mind and body. If we learn how to master our breath, we can open up energy gateways—or even ride the proverbial waves of the ebbs and flow of our lives.

Now there are a few things happening from an energetic level when we focus on breathing.

1. Our bodies are not stagnant, because they have to get off of their chairs, and that is when energy momentum starts. Newton's law of motion states: "A stationary object remains at rest until you apply a force to it. Once you set it in motion, the object continues to move at a constant speed until it strikes another object."

2. Once our bodies are outside, they are breathing fresh air, not recirculated air conditioned air; and God knows when was the last time the facilities manager changed the air filter!

3. Our bodies are taking deep breaths.

Remember that we talked about the importance of posture and how slouching would drain our energy? When we take deep breaths, our body posture physically has to change.

For a quick exercise, try this for yourself:

- Hunch over as much as you can.
- Then take deep breaths from your nose and try to fill up all of your stomach and lungs, while holding the bad posture as much as you can.

Now try this instead:

- Throw your shoulders back, and lift up your chest and your chin.
- Now try to take a deep breath through your nose, and fill up your belly and lungs.

In which exercise is it easier for you to breathe? Does air seem easier to take in as you are standing tall?

There are simple and powerful ways to change your posture, move your body, and take deep breaths to get your energy moving. When you consciously and consistently breathe, you will see a dramatic change in your energetic level. And when you combine breathing with the next energy booster, it will help get your energy to the next level.

CHAPTER 3

Third Energy Booster: Water

*"The simple truth is that dehydration can cause disease.
Everyone knows that water is 'good' for the body,
yet we seem not to know how it is to one's well-being."*

— Batmanghelidj, MD

Chronic dehydration is more common than you think. CBS Miami reported in their segment "Chronic Dehydration More Common Than You Think," on July 2, 2013, that 75 percent of Americans might suffer from chronic dehydration, according to doctors. We have all heard about the importance of drinking water and how we can survive two weeks without food, but we would die within a week if we didn't drink water.

The third key cornerstone to health and vitality is water, but there is more than just hydration to consider. Most people don't even realize how crucial water is to our health and vitality.

First, let's discuss how water heals your body, and second, why drinking water at the wrong time or temperature can zap the energy away from you.

Let me share with you a story about Dr. Fereydoon Batmanghelidj. Dr. Batmanghelidj is the author of the book *Your Body's Many Cries for Water*. He is also an internationally known researcher and advocate of the natural healing power of water. He studied under the Nobel Prize winner, Sir Alexander Fleming, who shared the discovery of penicillin. In 1979, the Iranian Revolution broke out, and Dr. B became a political prisoner. During the two years and seven months that he was in the infamous Evin Prison, one of the fellow prisoners came to Dr. B with crippling peptic ulcer pain. Without any medication available to the prisoners, Dr. B could only offer the patient two glasses of water. Within less than ten minutes, the patient's pain went away. Dr. B instructed the patient to drink two glasses of water every three hours. His patient became pain free for his four remaining months in Evin. Dr. B went on and successfully treated more than three thousand inmates with water, and Evin Prison proved to be an ideal "stress laboratory." Despite Dr. B being offered an earlier release, he chose to stay an extra four months to finish his research on dehydration and bleeding peptic ulcer disease, which was later published by *The New York Times* on June 21, 1983.

There are also research findings and evidence that drinking water can be amazingly helpful in treating many diseases—including rheumatoid arthritis pain, lower back pain, neck pain, angina pain, headaches, stress and depression, high blood pressure, higher blood cholesterol, excess body weight, asthma, allergies, diabetes, and dyspeptic pain. Every living organism on this planet is alive because of water. Drinking adequate amounts of water every day gives us more energy and helps us fight diseases. Ideally, you'll want to drink about six to eight ounces of water a day, depending on your level of activity. If you are an active person and work out a lot, you'll want to have more water intake. A general rule of thumb is to drink water before you get thirsty.

What most of us don't know is when to drink water and at what temperature to drink it. Let me ask you this. When you go to a restaurant, what does your waiter first bring you after you sit down at a table? Water, right? I know this sounds absurd, but that's how we have been conditioned to drink water: with our meals. According to traditional Chinese medicine, however, drinking during a meal dilutes our saliva and gastric juices in our stomachs—leading to poor digestion.

When we drink water, beer, OJ, and other liquids with our food, they water down the digestive enzymes in our body. In addition, drinking water during a meal causes the blood to become too concentrated. When our blood becomes too concentrated, it draws water from the cells around it.

In addition, according to traditional Chinese medicine, digestion is the key treatment to any illness. When our guts are operating correctly, meaning we are disseminating our waste properly and eating health food, we gain our health back. It all starts with water and not reducing the potency of our natural digestive enzymes.

Digestive enzymes help break down food that we eat into nutrients and enable us to digest food properly through our intestines—delivering nutrients into our bloodstream. These special proteins also help create chemicals to get rid of our waste, detox our blood, and empower our immune systems to fight against diseases. However, most of us are enzyme deficient, because when we drink coffee, consume white sugar, or eat processed food, it drains our enzyme sources.

Imagine for a moment that our digestion is an oven. When we eat food, we need to have fire in our stomachs to properly burn off the food. If the oven is on too high, the food that we eat flash burns in our stomachs, and we can't absorb the food. If our stomach fire is weak, then we can't properly digest the food in it. Bad digestion leads to most diseases, chronic aches and pains in our joints, and even weight gain!

When our enzyme levels deplete, our bodies ask our immune systems to help sustain digestion; that in return puts an additional strain on our immune systems to defend against diseases or illnesses. In addition, joint pain, food allergies, gout, and extreme fatigue can be caused by low enzyme reserves.

On the flip side, high levels of enzymes speeds up our digestive process, boosts our immune systems, helps us absorb nutrients better, and save us energy for other needs.

What else zaps our enzymes?

Go back to the water at the restaurant. What is in the water? Ice is in the water, right? Our bodies try really hard to maintain homeostasis or balance. There is a reason why our bodies are held constant at 98.6 degrees, not 102.1 or 94.5. Any slight deviation from our normal body temperature, and we go into hyperthermia as our brain cells fry from overheating; or we go into hypothermia as our nervous systems and organs stop functioning, and we go into shock.

So what should we do?

- Ideally, drink room temperature water, if not warm water. If you ever travel to Asia, restaurants serve warm water or warm tea, even if it's 100 degrees outside.
- Drink a glass of water first thing in the morning before you eat anything to cleanse your digestive track.
- Drink ten minutes before, or ideally thirty minutes before, your meal. The positive side effect of this practice is that drinking water before a meal will fill you up and stops you from overeating.
- Avoid drinking liquid ten minutes, or ideally thirty minutes, after your meal.

CHAPTER 4

How and When Do You Use the Abundance Energy Exercises to Help Yourself to Stay on Top of Your Game?

"You will never change your life until you change something you do daily. The secret of your success is found in your daily routine."

— Darren Hardy

Business Insider published an article on May 4, 2011, titled, "Why Successful People Leave Work Early." It turns out that the harder that we work without a break, the more we drive ourselves to the ground—and our productivity decreases exponentially.

Psychologist Dr. K. Anders Ericsson published a study in the *Psychological Review* discussing how successful people work harder in short bursts. They don't get distracted by multitasking or by checking emails every five seconds, and they don't answer all phone calls. In other words, they focus on what they are doing, and just as importantly, they allow themselves to take scheduled breaks.

When we take scheduled breaks, we reset our minds so that we come back to work later fresh. When we take a five to ten minute mental break after working for forty-five minutes, our brains come back refreshed and ready to knock out another round. I know multimillionaire entrepreneurs that have installed an alarm on their laptops, and at every forty-five minute mark, the alarm goes off and they take a quick mental break.

During those mental breaks, there are specific exercises to reset your brain and body and recharge your energy. We will explore those shortly.

From my personal experience, one of the major success factors contributing to why I was able to beat my sales quotas year over year as an account manager was that I took pauses during the day. I would stay extremely focused for forty-five minutes to one hour. That means no checking Facebook or email or anything that distracted me from work. Then, I would get up walk around after an hour to move and do the exercises I'm about to teach you.

Try taking breaks. You'll be surprised how much more productive you'll be. Although I would be on a roll plowing through work and sometimes passing the seventy-five minute mark, I would still force myself to peel my butt of the chair to take a five to ten minute break. Those short pauses don't seem like much, but five minute pauses throughout the day yield big energy returns.

During my short breaks, I also reminded myself to drink water to help my body, which had so many benefits. First, my brain stayed hydrated so that my brain could continue to process complex problems and tasks. Second, drinking water saved me from having back pain.

"Say what?!?"

As strange as it may seem, drinking water forced me to get up and visit the other office, the men's restroom. To be exact, it was the getting out of the chair, walking, and getting my body moving that saved me from back pain, because our bodies were never designed to sit hours on end.

I attend several Tony Robbins' live seminars with five thousand-plus attendees, and Tony frequently asks, "How many of you in this room suffer from back pain?" On average, one-third of the audience members raise their hands.

I will show you in the next section how to alleviate back pain. For the time being, the best that you can do is to get out of your chair and walk.

ACTION STEP EXERCISES

*Jump Start Your Energy with these Energy Rich Exercises
(refer to Energy Rich Workbook):*

*Exercise a: Creating the Perfect Posture
Exercise b: Unwinding to Allow Your Energy to Flow
Exercise c: Boosting Your Energy Meridian*

Get your hands on the Secret Energy Hack Section I —
Jump Start Your Own Energy Naturally.

DOWNLOAD your FREE bonus
Energy Exercise Workbook. Go to
www.allanting.com/IEMBookBonuses

**Remember, knowledge is not enough. Knowledge +
Action = Power! It only takes 5 minutes!**

Game Changer Questions

"Personal power is the ability to take action."

— Tony Robbins

1. What is the one thing you learned from "The Jump Start Your Own Energy Naturally" section that stood out the most for you today? It could be something new or a good reminder to reinforce what you already know.

2. In the last three months, what has your energy level been like on average? From a scale of 1 to 10, with 1 being super low energy and 10 being peak energy, where do you consistently live day in and day out?

3. On a regular basis, how do you portray yourself? Do you feel like your posture, voice, and energy are representing the person you want the world to see? Why is that? If you could be even better, what must you do differently?

Now that you know how to generate energy rich state naturally, it does no good if you don't know how to contain it. It would be like pumping air into a tire with a big hole in it. In the next section, we'll talk about what drains your energy and how to plug those holes so that you can retain your energy rich state.

What Are the Top Five Energy Drainers – *DRAIN?*

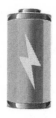

Diet Intake
Release Stress
Activities and Non-Movement
Identify Toxins
Negative Language Patterns

Secret Energy Hack Section II Overview

"Take care of your body with steadfast fidelity. The soul must see through these eyes alone and if they are dim, the whole world is clouded."

— Johann Wolfgang Von Geothe

In the last section, we explored how using your POW (Posture, Oxygen, Water) Instant Energy Method on a regular and consistent basis can help you generate the energy rich state at your fingertips. Now that we know how to generate the energy rich state, we must learn how to *retain* the energy that we generated.

Imagine you go to the gas station to pump air into your tire, but there is a hole in the tire you don't know about. No matter how much air you give to the tire, it will always be flat.

It's the same for your body. If you don't plug those energy draining holes, low energy can affect other areas of your life—such as your relationships, finances, work performance, and health.

Have you ever had only a couple hours of sleep, followed by a long day of work, which left you feeling overwhelmed and burnt out? I mean the type of day when you're stressed out to the max and at your limit.

That happens even to high performers at some point in their lives. As Type A achievers, most of them are multitasking to the max in this fast paced, busy society—and many of them are stressed to their limits.

When we are stressed out or burnt out, we typically are operating at Quadrant 3, Energy Poor and Exhaustion. This is a very dangerous quadrant to be in. Often we don't know where our stress limit is, and we are a ticking time bomb waiting to explode.

Quadrant 1 Energy Rich Energy Lasting	Quadrant 2 Energy Rich Energy Non-Lastiing
Quadrant 3 Energy Poor Exhaustion	Quadrant 4 Energy Poor Lethargic

When we are operating with limited energy, others may look at us the wrong way or say something that we disagree with, and we explode and let them have it. It doesn't help when our fuse is already short, does it?

Or let me ask you this: if you were to recall an argument that you had with your colleague, a friend, or a loved one recently, and break down exactly how you felt, what would you say?

- Would you say that maybe you felt *frustrated?*
- Did you feel *irritated?*
- How about *uncertain, angry, tense,* or *stressed out?*
- Maybe it was *all of the above?*
- How about your *energy level?*
- Did you feel *energy rich* or *energy poor?*
- Did you feel *more open* or *more closed?*

Most would say that when they are running low on energy and experience unnecessary conflict in a key relationship, they feel irritated, angry, heavy, and closed off. When we get into a closed and irritated state, the battle is already lost, because we're not open to any alternative solutions. We unfortunately become *pig-headed,* don't we?

I know this well, because this happened to me twelve years ago. I was at a fast-paced technology start-up company working twelve hour days. I also had a three hour commute back and forth every day. Our team was under a lot of pressure to deliver a $500,000 project. Because of mismanagement, however, we discovered that we were not going to be able to deliver the project on time and within budget. Our VP called for a staff meeting, and she was really upset at us for not meeting the project deadline.

To add to the stress level, our company announced a 50 percent workforce reduction, and many of my friends at work were let go. There was so much uncertainty with employment that I didn't know if I would have a job in the next thirty days.

I left work feeling angry and stressed out—and all of my energy just drained out of me. I came home that night and had dinner with my then-girlfriend. During the middle of our meal, we got in a huge fight.

The argument was so stupid. I couldn't believe we argued about who was going to wash the dishes. Does this sound familiar? Have you ever gotten into an argument about who is going to do the chores or something similar that is really petty? Sure, we have all.

I got angry, I yelled at her, I stormed out of the apartment, and I slammed the door as hard as I could. My patience *ran out*, because I was so *stressed out*. I was at an energy poor state—angry and bitter. To this day, this sensation is something I absolutely hate. I hate the feeling when the pressure from work is affecting my personal life, and I feel like I have no way out.

As I am sharing this story with you, I am sure I am only talking about myself, and you've never gotten into a heated argument with someone you love, right?

Had I known what were the top five energy drainers, I would have been able to manage my low energy more effectively. I would not have felt as irritated, frustrated, or angry when talking to my girlfriend. Instead, I would have had more patience and talked to her more calmly.

In this section, I will discuss *the top five energy drainers that will suck the energy out of you so* that you don't let low energy affect your life, your career, your finances, and your loved ones.

Here is a simple acronym to remember those energy drainers by – DRAIN

- **D**iet Intake
- **R**elease Stress
- **A**ctivity and Non-Movement
- **I**dentify Toxins
- **N**egative Language Patterns

Let's dive right into what is draining your energy.

CHAPTER 5

Diet Intake

"You can have it all...Just not all at once."

— Oprah Winfrey

D o you remember your last Thanksgiving dinner? Was there a big turkey in the center of the table? Did it have stuffing inside? Can you still smell the turkey? Was there a big plate of mashed potatoes? Did Mom make her favorite casserole? Can you still taste the big and round pumpkin pie?

Yummy, right? Don't tell me you aren't already salivating...

Let's break down a typical Thanksgiving dinner. We all gather around for dinner, and every inch of our dining table is covered with plates. The classic Thanksgiving meal includes a 15-pound turkey; a sauce plate with dark, gooey beef gravy; a plate for stuffing; another plate for cranberries; a big bowl of garlic mashed potatoes; a dish for the green bean casserole; and a basket of biscuits. In the distant corner, we have something healthy: a bowl of green leaf salad.

The feast begins as we start piling up the food on our plates. When we finally stuff ourselves with enough turkey, stuffing, and mashed potatoes, "us guys" grab our belts, open them, and loosen them a couple of notches so that we can let our stomachs expand and breathe.

It doesn't stop there. Mom comes around and asks, "Who wants pumpkin pie?" Even though we've totally stuffed ourselves with food (and now resemble the turkey!), we still say, "Yeah, Mom, I'll have some pie! Oh, by the way, do we have vanilla ice cream to go with it?"

After we shove down the pie, we go look for a landing area. That is typically the living room couch or the Lazy Boy 2000. We lie on the sofa, feeling exhausted and pooped out. We ate so much that we became the stuffed turkey. This is the classic stage for the food coma to begin its drama.

Overeating doesn't just happen on Thanksgiving. Have you ever eaten a big chili cheeseburger with garlic fries at lunch and come back to work feeling groggy and tired? When you go into a 2 p.m. business meeting, your eyelids get heavy, and you start to nod your head as you fall asleep? I'm sure many of us have experienced something similar.

When we eat one hundred times more than the amount our bodies ever need, the majority of our blood directs toward our stomachs for digestion, which means we have lot a less blood directed towards our brains and other vital organs. *No wonder we have low energy!* So avoid eating heavy meals if you want more energy in your life!

And by the way, Elvis Presley's personal physician, Dr. Nick, released the book, *The King and Dr. Nick: What Really Happened to Elvis and Me.* It talked about how Elvis didn't really die from cardiac arrhythmia. Dr. Nick revealed from the autopsy that "…Presley's colon was 5 to 6 inches in diameter (whereas the normal width is 2 to 3 inches), and instead of being the standard 4 to 5 feet long, his colon was 8 to 9 feet in length."

So what should we eat instead? We'll cover foods that boost energy in the next section.

CHAPTER 6

Release Stress

"Cortisol: Why 'The Stress Hormone' Is Public Enemy No. 1."
— Psychology Today

We have talked about stress from a mindset perspective, so let's dive deeper into how stress affects our physical bodies and our immune systems.

I was at a technology summit recently and overheard two professionally dressed women talking about how every employee at a very well-known tech company goes through a serious mental breakdown during their first year of employment. The women laughed and said, "That is a part of their rite of passage working there." Let me ask you:

- Have you ever had a hard time sleeping at night, because you were obsessing about work?
- Do you have a habit of checking your smartphone before you sleep to make sure you have caught up with all of your emails?
- Do you have a habit of running to Starbucks or your local barista in the morning to get a *ginormous* size of macchiato with two shots of espresso—no foam and less water? And before having your coffee, do you feel like a zombie because

you didn't sleep well the night before and the coffee is the only thing that gets you going?

I know how you feel, because I've been there too. When we get to the office, we are multitasking from one project to another. We respond to more emails and attend meeting after meeting. After work, we have to pick up the kids from school and drop them off at soccer practice. Then we have to go to Whole Foods to pick up groceries. The to-do list goes on and on...

Then we are checking our emails again at 11:30 p.m., and we fall right back into the vicious cycle from the night before. This happens day in and day out, until one day, we hit the proverbial wall—the stress limit.

So how do we know if we're hitting the stress limit? Here are tell-tale signs of stress.

Have you ever:

- Felt agitated, frustrated, and moody?
- Felt overwhelmed, like you're losing control or need to take control?
- Had a hard time relaxing and quieting your mind?
- Ground your teeth at night?
- Experienced low energy, headaches, upset stomach, or insomnia?

If you have experienced any of the above, chances are you have had stress related symptoms. The problem is that stress overflows into our everyday lives and causes havoc to our relationships, decreases job performance, and diminishes our well-being—as evidenced when I lost my cool and flipped out at my girlfriend.

Let's break stress down and see how it affects our bodies, our immune systems, and our well-being. The stress state is also known as the *flight or fight or sympathetic* state, and we are experiencing this more than ever in our lives. Whenever we are stressed out, we are firing off biochemicals in our heads called cortisol or stress hormones. Long term exposure to higher than normal levels of cortisol makes us age faster, causes adrenal fatigue, and negatively affects our immune systems. Because we are constantly on the run and multitasking in our modern daily lives, our brains barely get a chance to rest.

So how does the constant firing of cortisol in your brain affect you in the long run? You don't have to be medical doctor or hold a clinical PhD to know this, but if I were to ask you what part of your body system gets prioritized if you were to be chased by a saber-toothed tiger, what would you say? I mean, imagine you are fighting for your life; which part of your body system has to be activated in order to survive?

Your adrenal system must kick in to heighten your senses, right? How about your muscular system and respiratory system—to help keep you in the fight to stay alive?

On the flipside, which part of your system becomes secondary? Do you need to focus on your digestion right now? Do you need to process the food in your stomach? Of course not! How about your reproductive system? Do you feel like you must reproduce right now? No, of course not. You're about to die at the jaws of a tiger! You don't have time to reproduce!

In the fast paced, modern world, we constantly stress out for prolonged periods of time, and that is why stress is linked to many modern diseases and conditions—including heart failure, diabetes, asthma, ulcers, and many more. And what do we do after we are finally done with tasks from work, the to do list, and dinner? Do we go for a walk and clear the clutter in our minds? No, we sit on the couch and turn on our TVs. Did you know that the average American watches more than six hours of TV a day, according to Nielsen Ratings? In an average adult lifespan, one would have used more than sixteen years watching TV. At the minimum wage of $7.25 an hour, we would have lost $1,013,550 in our lifetime.

What is worse is that TV is designed to stimulate our brains. If you didn't already know it, most TV news channels are designed to broadcast negative news, because what they care about is Nielsen Ratings. The higher the rating, the more commercials they can air and sustain their business. News media know how to boost their viewer ratings. They use bad news to hook people into their news stories.

Let's do a simple experiment. Let's take a walk on Market Street in downtown San Francisco on a Monday morning. As you are walking past one of the green newspaper kiosks, you notice a headline from the *San Francisco Chronicle* in bold that says, "Top geophysicist pinpoints next big earthquake in San Francisco today." Would you:

a) Keep walking or
b) Stop by and grab the newspaper to find out more?

My bet is b, because your brain is hardwired to identify threats so that you can survive.

The next time you turn on CNN (let's call it Cable Negative News), count the number of negative news stories to positive news stories. I bet you'll be surprised at the ratio.

Don't let stress take hostage of your life. Don't drown in the waves. Learn how to surf with the tide. We'll learn specific strategies and exercises on how to overcome stress towards the end of this section.

CHAPTER 7

Activity and Non-Movement

The 21ˢᵗ Century Lifestyle

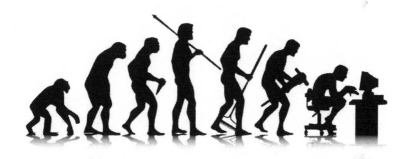

I taught at Yahoo recently and asked my students, "How many of you sit on a chair for hours on end?" Just about everyone raised their hands. I then asked them, "How many of you have experienced back pain?" I got a range between 40 to 60 percent of people raising their hands.

Unfortunately, this isn't true just at Yahoo. I have asked the same exact questions at HP, Amazon, eBay, and Microsoft—and about the same percentage of employees raised their hands.

In the twenty-first century, many of us live stagnant, non-active, and what I call *"boxed up" lives.* We wake up in a box. We box our breakfast. We drive a box to work. We work in a box cube. We type on a box. We have a boxed lunch. We drive our box home. We make our dinner from a box package. We turn on a box screen to watch our favorite program.

No wonder sometimes we feel trapped and boxed in! It's because we live in a box, and we don't move. The human body simply was not built to sit for so many hours each day. Thousands of years ago, our ancestors were hunters and migrant people who moved around from one water source to another, hunting and gathering berries. We were active—building fire and creating shelters to survive.

When we knew how to grow our own food sources, we became farmers in an agricultural society—growing grains, vegetables, and fruits. We were still in motion using our picks, axes, and buffaloes to plow our land. We would get up early at sunrise and go to sleep as the sun went down.

As we progressed into the industrial age, we started to move less and less. We worked in factory assembly lines, putting together parts to assemble the Ford Model T.

However, in the information age, and for the first time ever in human history, today we sit in office chairs, behind desks, in front of our computers. Combine this with bad posture, and it's no wonder we have low energy. Our bodies were never designed to sit hours on end.

Let's do a quick self-assessment:

- On average, how many hours do you sit a day—three hours, five hours, eight hours a day?
- Have you ever seen someone's shoulder hiked up so far that her shoulder is almost up to the jaw line—like a turtle hiding inside its shell?
- Did you ever massage your own shoulders to relieve the neck and shoulder pain?

- Would you like to know why we get a tight neck and shoulders?

Let's use the cartoon caveman Fred Flintstone as an example. Back in cartoon dinosaur days, when a saber-toothed tiger chased Fred, he either jumped into his foot pedaling vehicle with Barney to run away, or he stood and fought the tiger with his big, brown wooden club.

Let me ask you this. When the saber-toothed tiger opens its jaws and spreads its 4-inch fangs, which part of the prey does it go after? The prey's left leg? The prey's arm? Or does the tiger go after the carotid artery?

It instinctively goes to the neckline for the kill, right? So physiology wise, when we're in the fight or flight state, we hike up our shoulders to protect our neckline.

You might be saying, "You know, the odds of us confronting a saber-toothed tiger are slim these days. That means the fight or flight syndrome doesn't really apply to us, right?" Not really. Whenever we are stressed out, we are firing off the same cortisol over and over again, and our body doesn't gets a chance to rest.

If we were to take a time lapse photo of our shoulders from the beginning of the day to the end of the day, we'd see a big difference. Our shoulders would be higher than when we started. This phenomenon has to do with the fight or flight response. Our body reacts to daily stress just like it would in the saber-toothed tiger story that I just shared.

In the future, if you're stressed out, just throw your shoulders back to change your posture, and take a minute or so to take a few rounds of deep breaths.

CHAPTER 8

Identify Toxins: Eliminate or Dramatically Reduce Acid Addictions

"We are digging our graves with our teeth."

— Thomas Moffett

For the longest time, I couldn't get rid of my love handles—the fat around my belly. I tried cardio workouts five times a week. I went to the gym every day to lift weights. I also did P90X for three months. If you're not familiar with P90X, it's a very intense program that has you working out every day of the week for three months straight. I also watched my diet and ate according to the P90X suggestions.

Although I dropped 20 pounds in three months and saw drastic changes in my body, I still had a layer of love handle fat around my stomach. I thought it was just my genetics and how I was built, so I accepted my body.

However, I was wrong. I completed an eight day health retreat in Fiji where I did a four day liquid fast. For food, all we consumed was water, two bowls of hot ginger soup, two glasses avocado smoothie, and five shots omega 3 and omega 6 oils. As a part of my cleanse option, I did five sessions of colonics, where I went to a hydro colon therapy facility to clean out my bowel and colon.

At the end of the fifth day, I jumped on the scale at the clinic for fun, and what happened next shocked me. I had lost another five pounds. I ran back to my room, got in front of the bathroom mirror, took my shirt off, and looked at my belly. The love handle that was there before was now gone! I couldn't believe my eyes. I had gotten rid of excess waste and toxins in my body, and my skin was glowing.

I was able to lose the fat around my belly, because I was able to cleanse and release the toxins in my body through the liquid fast and hydro colon therapy. I know I didn't lose "water weight," because I had been drinking liquids all day long. Although I didn't eat anything for four days, I had more energy than before—and I had pretty good energy to begin with.

It turns out that when our bodies get rid of the toxins, the fat goes away too. One of the fat's primary functions is to help insulate our bodies from poisons and block the toxins from doing further damage to our bodies. So when I released the toxins out of my body, the fat went along with it.

So chances are if you're overweight or would like to lose some fat around your belly or thighs, it's not a fat problem. Most likely it's a problem with the acid level in your body. When your body is not pH balanced—such as when you have too much acid in your body—two things happen:

1. Your body will likely produce more insulin, causing you to store more fat, and
2. The acid will cause your cells to break down, because your pancreas is over stimulated with insulin.

In Chinese Medicine, 99 percent of treatment of any disease starts with the digestive tract. When you clean your digestive system, you have a foundation upon which to fight off other diseases and viruses. It's ideal to do a liquid cleanse at least once a year or twice a year to get rid of the pollution in your body, so that you feel more energy. The best time to do a cleanse is in the spring when the weather is warm, if not during the summer—because it's less demanding on your system than during the winter cold weather. Just like you get a routine oil change for your car, you need to do routine preventive maintenance for your body.

During the four-day cleanse, some of the participants were having major headaches and feeling nauseated. Those who felt sick mostly came from having a bad diet or a bad lifestyle. One person in our group in particular was a medical doctor. She had been taking a sleeping pill on a regular basis, because she worked a night shift and couldn't sleep during the day. She felt sick throughout the entire first part of the liquid cleanse. On the fourth day, she flushed out the toxins in her body and felt so much better. She had more energy, her headaches went away, and her skin was glowing once she eliminated the toxins in her body.

"Let food be thy medicine and medicine be thy food."
— Hippocrates

In this section, we are going to define the major culprits of why more than one-third of Americans are obese and why we spend $147 billion annually on medical care. In addition, obesity isn't just about being overweight anymore. It's also about being ill. Obesity-related conditions include type-2 diabetes, cancer, heart disease, and stroke.

When we eat or intake mostly acid based foods or beverages like TV dinners, packaged foods, and Coke, we are promoting the growth of bacteria, fungus, yeast, and viruses that break down our cells and tissues in our body.

It's like this. Have you ever seen the movie *Grumpy Old Men* where John threw some fish in the back of Max's car, and in a few days, Max's car smelled like something was decaying, and he was disgusted with the rotten smell? It's because the fish cells began to deteriorate from growing bacteria that evolved into yeast and mold. That same reaction is happening inside your body when you over consume acid based foods and drinks.

Have you ever smelled someone with bad breath? Did that awful smell reminds you of something decaying? Well that is how degenerative and infectious diseases begin in our body.

Toxin #1: Sugar Pie Honey Bunch

The American Heart Association says that the amount of sugar we eat has a direct association with heart disease, cancer, poor sleep quality, depression, acne, infertility, impotence, and high blood pressure. Dr. Mark Hyman, a regular blog contributor on *Huffington Post*, even referenced sugar to illegal drugs. Actually, that's not too far from the truth. When we consume high-sugar foods like breakfast cereal, you know the ones with cartoon characters on the boxes, our brains light up like a Christmas tree on an MRI machine. The part of our brain that responds to cocaine or heroin is the same one that reacts to sugar.

We as Americans are leading the consumption of sugar in the world, and we are consuming more than ever in the history of human existence. The average American consumes about 130 pounds of sugar a year. In 1900, the average was less than 60 pounds a year.

Recently, a documentary called *Fed Up* debuted in movie theaters, which talks about how the food industry is actually creating more havoc to our health rather than helping our well-being. One of the major focuses in the movie is about the increase in sugar consumption and how it's leading to the worldwide epidemic of obesity.

In the documentary, filmmakers Katie Couric and Laurie David have challenged the public to the "Fed Up Challenge" to give up all types of sugar for ten days. Even Kim Kardashian is jumping on board with the challenge.

Now it's not easy to identify sugar, even when the packaging looks healthy and branding refers to the product as organic. These hidden sugar names include sucrose, agave, or evaporated cane sugar. So always read the labels in the back of the packaged food.

My advice? Stay away from packaged food as much as possible. If you see the 150 ingredients in the packaging label and words you can't even pronounce like monosodium glutamate, maltodextrin, sodium caseinate, and autolyzed yeast, don't eat it! Do you ever see any of those additives on the labels of fresh kale, broccoli, and wheatgrass? Of course not! So eat freshly grown vegetables—organic if possible—directly from what is grown from the ground.

Now if I were to ask you which item has more sugar, a Twinkie or an organic peanut butter and jelly sandwich, which one would you choose? To give you an idea how much sugar is in a PB&J, we would have to eat three and a half Twinkies to equal the amount of sugar—even if the raspberry jam is organic—because the first ingredient in the jam is evaporated cane juice (AKA sugar).

In the next few years, I believe that the FDA should demand warning labels be put on processed food, just as the FDA has regulated the cigarette industry. As a nation, we are so addicted to sugar, and out of proportion with our consumption of it, that the world's leading cola brand contains more sugar than the World Health Organization recommends we consume in a day. Oh, and the cola cans/bottles keep getting bigger! By the way, one 12 ounce can of cola has more sugar than two Frosted Pop Tarts and a Twinkie combined!

Also avoid high fructose corn syrup and processed, highly refined sugar. Get rid of colas, and don't start your morning with sugar based cereals, because sugar will spike your insulin and dopamine, and by mid morning, your body will crave the same sugar rush level you gave it in the morning. Don't sail off your day with cartoon captain cereal. He'll have you shipwrecked in the long run!

Toxin #2: Coffee, The Expensive Emperor's New Coat

Do you know what is the world's second most value commodity behind petroleum? It's coffee beans. More than four hundred billion cups of coffee are served every year worldwide, and we Americans love to spend more than $1,000 per year on coffee. It's a very expensive emperor's coat, if you're looking for caffeine to boost your energy to get your day going.

In fact, besides being expensive, if your end goal is to get more energy in your life, drinking coffee is probably one of the worst strategies. This is even more true if you are sleep deprived—meaning if you average less than six hours of sleep a day.

Yeah, you might be saying, "I want to be even more productive in my life, and I'll have plenty of time to sleep when I'm dead! I have so many things that need to get done. My morning vanilla latte from Starbucks will help me get going."

Since we're on the topic of fables here, remember the old fable, "The Goose that Lays the Golden Egg?" That applies here as well. You might increase your productivity 10 percent to 90 percent day by drinking coffee, but you'll wreck your body if you continue doing this in the long run.

Here is what actually is happening inside your brain when you drink coffee. Picture for a moment that your energy is like a bank, and you are maxed out at $100. When you deplete your energy down to $20, you start to feel tired and want a recharge, so you reach for a venti double shot espresso, extra foam. The caffeine will bring you back to baseline level, because your brain is basically tricking you into thinking you have more energy. You'll feel invigorated, more alive, and eager to do things—but that's only your perception. In reality, the energy you perceive is really an optical illusion.

What is really happening inside your brain is a chemical reaction called adenosine triphosphate (ATP) breaking down into adenosine. Adenosine is what releases energy inside your brain. When this biochemical reaction is all over and you're stuck with only adenosine and no ATP left, the adenosine hits your nerve cells to make you tired, thus telling you to slow down. You know when you barely can keep your eyes open at work, but instead— what do you do? You go reach for more coffee, and you feel like you're back on the throne and in charge again. Well, kind of. You may feel like you have more energy, but you don't have as much as you could with the *higher level of energy* version of yourself.

I'm about to reveal the invisible emperor's new clothes. The trick about caffeine is, it fits where adenosine fits, so it blocks the feeling of being tired. Now that works during the short term, but the detrimental part of it is, you're not giving your body a chance to replenish your energy molecules. You might not feel tired, because you are just borrowing against your energy bank reserves. In reality, however, you only have so much energy capacity at that point.

Going back to the energy bank example, drinking coffee is like using your credit card when you are already in debt. You really want to buy the $10,000 Burberry Prorsum Hand-painted Shearling & Suede Trench Coat, but you only make $3,000 ($100 a day times thirty days) a month, so you just keep using your credit card. You buy the coat, but it's going to cost you a whole lot more later on.

If you run an energy deficit all of the time by not getting a consistent seven to nine hours of sleep per day—*and* you drink coffee—you are beating a dead horse to force more energy out of yourself. That debt keeps mounting higher and higher, and it impairs your productivity. When the amount of debt is so high, you do not have the molecules to be attentive and focused. You don't feel tired, because your perception is that you're performing well. But it's far from reality, because you don't have the energy producing chemicals in your brain. Even though you feel like you're amped up, it's not productive, useful energy you experience.

What we really need is recovery time—by getting a consistent, good night's sleep to redeposit ATP into our energy bank accounts and prime our cells for future use. When you do that, you'll be more productive at work. You'll have more energy in your life. You'll be happier. You might even get promoted and make more money to afford the new Burberry coat and a pair of $2,000 LV shoes to go with it.

Want to know about a coffee hack and how to cheat your system? When you stop drinking coffee for a long period of time, you can use coffee to temporarily boost your energy level. When I worked at large, high tech companies, we used to have to attend four day annual conferences in Las Vegas. The challenge was: how I do I party until four a.m. while being ready to attend the breakout sessions at eight a.m.? You guessed it, I drank coffee to stay awake and cheat my system. There is a caveat though. Although I was physically present, it didn't mean that I was mentally there. My mind was still in La-La Land, dreaming of sheep jumping over fences. The other caveat is this only works if you are not a regular coffee drinker.

Toxin #3: Cigarettes, *The Insider*

The harmful effects of cigarettes are pretty blatant. If you haven't seen the movie, *The Insider*, with Al Pacino and Russell Crowe, I highly recommend it. It covers a whistleblower in the tobacco industry bringing down the seven dwarfs of tobacco companies in 1994. In 2014, 159,260 people died from lung cancer, and 224,210 new cases of lung cancer were reported.

You might be thinking, "Yeah, I already know why smoking is bad for me," but maybe there is a lesson learned here.

When I graduated from college, I got a job working as a consultant implementing software projects. When I was going through PeopleSoft training with my new colleagues, we noticed a pattern with our practice director. The more stressed out he got, the more visits to the first floor patio he took to get his cigarettes breaks. Heck, he even held a chalk like a cigarette when he gave us a presentation, and he almost smoked the chalk at one point in his talk.

Smokers know this well. *What do smokers do when they are stressed out to calm themselves down?* They get up from their desks and take a walk outside of the building. They reach for their lighter and cigarette. They put the cigarette in their mouths and light up with their lighter. What do they do to get their cigarettes lit up? They have to take deep, diaphragmatic breaths to get it going and keep inhaling to finish the cigarette. Remember in the last section when we talked about one of the most powerful ways to generate energy in our lives? *It's taking deep, conscious breaths.* Essentially that is what smokers are doing. You can manage your stress and energy without the cigarettes, however, and you will be better off.

Toxin #4: Alcohol, The Hangover

Years ago, my dad read an article from the newspaper saying that heart surgeons recommended drinking one glass of merlot a day for great vascular health, and so my dad started drinking more and more.

What often happens in the medical field is that the medical studies get siloed, and the rest of us hear about conflicting information. Although drinking alcohol may improve circulation, as I stated earlier in the book, the cardiovascular surgeons never talked to the brain doctors and neurosurgeons. Dr. Melvin Knisely, who has been nominated for the Nobel Prize several times said, "Every time a person takes one drink of alcohol—even a social one—he permanently damages his brain, killing off thousands of brain cells" (McLennan).

CHAPTER 9

Negative Language Patterns

"Every thought you are thinking creates a wave in the unified field.
It ripples through all the layers of intellect, mind, senses, and matter,
spreading out in wider and wider circles."

— Deepak Chopra

It turns out that negative thoughts affect your nervous system, your immune system, and your energy. In recent years, scientists found evidence that how we think affects our bodies. Dr. Richard J. Davidson, director of the University of Wisconsin Laboratory for the Affective Neuroscience, found that people who suffer from depression have a higher risk for heart disease and other illnesses. Their brains' prefrontal cortexes are associated with negative emotions that appear to weaken people's immune response to a flu vaccine (Goode).

But why do some only focus on negative things like how shitty their lives are when it's beautiful outside—sunny and 85 degrees? Or why do some people focus only on how something bad always happens to them? It's just like the character Jim Carrey played in the movie *Bruce Almighty*. He blamed God for all of the mishaps in his life. In one scene, Bruce walked right into a puddle of muddy water with his right foot. He pulled his foot out of the puddle;

stared at his soaked tennis shoe, sock, and pants; looked up with absolute disgust; and asked God, "Why, why?"

I watched a live version of the movie *Bruce Almighty* on a San Francisco municipal bus six months ago. My wife received a parking citation recently, and she wanted to contest her ticket at the municipal court. She had never taken public transportation before because she grew up in Sacramento, I decided to show her how to get around San Francisco on a bus. We hopped on the long, orange, caterpillar looking 38 Geary bus line and threw in our quarters at the metal money collection box. She saw an empty single person seat in the front of the bus, so she walked past the other seated passengers to sit. Usually the front row seats on buses are reserved for elderly or disabled people, but since she was two months pregnant and the bus wasn't crowded, I thought it was okay for her to sit there. I stood next to her, holding onto the grab bars on the ceiling of the bus, as I thumbed through my Google map on my iPhone to figure out which bus stop we need to get off on.

About fifteen minutes into the bus ride, a well dressed woman in her mid fifties with curly red hair walked up to my wife and demanded that she give up her seat. With her heavy European accent she scolded, "Get out of the seat. You can't sit here."

My wife—poor sweet girl—was totally confused, because the middle-aged woman was neither disabled nor old; but anyway, she stood up and let the woman have the seat. As she stood halfway up, the bus driver slammed on the brake to avoid a rear-end collision to another car, and my wife started flying towards the front of the bus. I instantly grabbed her right arm just in time before she fell, and during the process, she accidentally stepped on another passenger on the bus.

A few seconds later, we heard someone scream bloody murder. It was a scruffy homeless looking guy in his late forties wearing a black SF Giants baseball cap, holding his right foot with both of his hands. It turned out that while my wife was fumbling her way out of her seat, she accidently stepped on his beat-up, greasy old Adidas sneakers. My wife said, "I'm really sorry," to the grungy looking man, while the middle aged woman forced her way into the single person seat as if she was entitled to it.

My wife was trying to get her composure back to figure out what just went wrong, when the same man started shouting, "God, why are you doing this to me? God, what have I done to deserve this? Great, just great. It always happens to me. Thanks a lot!" It was followed by a bunch of F-bomb yelling at the Big Guy above.

I really wanted to laugh, because it was just like the character Jim Carrey played, as he blew everything out of proportion. But I bit my tongue, because I didn't want to pour holy water gasoline into his Fire God.

"What does God have to do with this?" I thought to myself. It was merely a mishap.

I reflected later and talked to my wife about the incident, because we are both students of human behavior and why people do the things they do. I asked her, "Why do some people feel like life is never fair to them or something bad always happens to them? Then you look at someone like Nick Vujicic who was born with no arms, no legs, and only one tiny left foot. Everything is a challenge in his life. If he wants to eat at the dinner table, he needs to climb to the top of the chair, using no arm and no legs. If he wants to get to the couch to watch TV, he needs to climb down the chair, hobble across the room, climb on the sofa, and use his mouth and teeth to turn on the TV."

How many of us would be somewhat resentful with the body that we got? Not Nick. He is happier than a clam. These physical limitations never stopped Nick from achieving his dreams. Instead, Nick goes around the world giving inspirational keynote speeches—sharing how he overcame his struggles. He is happily married with a beautiful wife and child.

The story of the homeless man on the 38 Geary bus is a classic example of someone playing the martyr role or the victim role. I'm mean, he's got two arms and two legs and is in relatively good health condition—unlike our friend Nick who struggles with the everyday basic motor skills that we take for granted, like using a fork to eat. Oh, and learning how to use chopsticks to eat sushi? Forget about it.

Do you know of someone who complains about life? Complains about a job? Complains about a relationship? Maybe that person was you? I know I've done it—plenty of it actually.

So how do we get out of this negative rut? Do we just think happy thoughts and never become angry? Do we drug ourselves through anti-depressant pills, do illegal drugs, overeat, or drown ourselves in alcohol? Do we just mentally check out and stop caring anymore?

These methods will provide temporary relief, but they are not an effective strategy. Now I'm not telling you just to say to yourself, "I'm happy. I'm happy. I'm happy." That might work for a while, but your happy thoughts would only go so far.

Instead, be aware of the questions you ask often. Not all questions that you ask are equal. Some questions dis-empower you. Some questions propel you to the next level. Generally "why" types of questions do you a disservice, because the quality and tone of your answer reflects the quality and tone of the question. If you ask yourself a disempowering question, you'll likely get a disempowering answer.

As an awareness exercise, ask yourself these questions, and jot down your answers:

- "What's wrong with me?"
- *Your answer:*
- "Why can't I learn this fast enough?"
- *Your answer:*
- "Why can't I lose weight?" or "Why am I so fat?"
- *Your answer:*
- "Why am I so unlucky?"
- *Your answer:*
- "Why am I such an idiot?"
- *Your answer:*

Have you ever asked these questions or similar questions? We have all done it. The fundamental problem with "why" type of questions is that these questions presuppose that there is something wrong. They really don't serve us.

Let's break down these questions: "What's wrong with me?" presupposes that there is something wrong. "Why can't I learn this fast enough?" presupposes that you are a slow learner. "Why can't I lose weight?" or "Why am I fat?" presupposes that "you can't lose weight and you are fat," and on and on...

Watch your brain focus on whatever you feed it. It won't tell you that you have asked a disempowering question. Instead, your brain will instinctively give you the answer that you ask. It's just like going to Google to ask, "Why am I so fat?" and you'll get answers from WebMD telling you that you eat too much.

Now what I'd like you to do is instead of asking "why" questions, ask more empowering ones. Answer these questions:

- "What's going well in my life?"
- *Your answer:*
- "What do I love most about myself?"
- *Your answer:*

- "What is the best weight loss strategy?"
- *Your answer:*
- "What can I be even more happy about today?"
- *Your answer:*

Now compare your answers with the previous answers you wrote down. What have you noticed is different? Do you get much better results with the empowering questions?

Be extra aware of the questions you ask yourself. If you're getting an answer you don't like, go back and ask yourself a better question to break the negative conversation and pattern.

Here are the daily empowering questions that I ask myself in the morning to start my day. These questions help me stay focused, dialed in, and on track with my goals. I especially use them when I feel like I'm spinning out of control, overwhelmed, angry, or frustrated—to help me get back to what matters most in my life:

1. **What could I be even more grateful about in my life right now?** Which area of my life makes me grateful? How does that make me feel?
2. **What could I be even happier about in my life right now?** Which area of my life makes me happy? How does that make me feel?
3. **What could I be even more excited about in my life right now?** Which area of my life makes me excited? How does that make me feel?
4. **What could I be even more proud of my life right now?** Which area of my life makes me proud? How does that make me feel?
5. **What could I enjoy even more in my life right now?** Which area of my life do I enjoy most? How does that make me feel?

6. **What is going *right* in my life right now?** Which area of my life makes me feel like I'm on track? How does that make me feel?

7. **Who do I love in my life, and who loves me?** How does that make me feel?

Take a few minutes each morning to answer at least one of these questions. Notice if you feel more centered, more excited, or more alive after answering these questions. These will help build your emotional muscles and make them stronger and stronger.

Plug the Energy Draining Holes Exercises:

So we talked about what not to do or the things to watch out for. Now let's talk about what to do—and the simple yet powerful strategies to plug the energy draining holes so that we can help you get out of Quadrant 3: Energy Poor, Exhaustion and towards Quadrants 1 and 2.

ACTION STEP EXERCISES

Ready to PLUG THE ENERGY DRAINING HOLES?

Go to the Section II of your *Energy Rich Workbook* now for the stress relief exercises. If you haven't got your workbook, go to **www.AllanTing.com/IEMBookBonuses** and **DOWNLOAD your FREE bonus Energy Exercise Workbook.**

Look under Secret Energy Hack Section II—What Drains Our Life Energy?

Plug the Energy Drainer Exercises (refer to Energy Rich Workbook):

Exercise a: Stress Relief
Exercise b: Neck Pain Relief
Exercise c: Back Pain Relief Part A
Exercise d: Back Pain Relief Part B

Game Changer Questions

"It is in your moments of decision that your destiny is shaped."
— Tony Robbins

1. What is the one thing that you learned in this section, which if you implemented, would change your life?
2. In which areas of your life do you feel overwhelmed, energy drained, stressed out, or exhausted on a regular basis?
3. If you became more committed to increasing your energy today—more than you ever have before—what would you *do* right now, and what would you stop doing immediately? Why is making this change a *must do* and not a *should do?*

Now that you know how to plug the energy draining holes, how do you continue to build the energy reservoir in your body, so that you have lasting energy—kind of like the Energizer battery bunny that keeps going and going? How do you have continuous energy for the long run? I'll share something that Oprah and Dr. Oz highly recommend to boost your immune system and your flow of vital energy.

That's all in the next section and keep up the hard work!

Manage Your Energy For Life

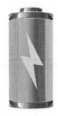

Qigong – Ancient Secret Chinese Energy Practice Top 7 Natural Foods to Sustain Your Quadrant 1, Energy Rich Energy Lasting State

Secret Energy Hack Section III Overview

"Life's a marathon, not a sprint."

— Dr. Phil

A friend of mine asked, "Why do I feel so burnt out and have low energy all the time?" He just couldn't figure it out. He shared his weekly exercise and eating routine with me, and it was impressive. At first glance, it looked like he was doing all the right things. But at closer glance, we uncovered some hitches.

Here was his weekly routine, and you tell me if his exercise program was sustainable—meaning that he could do this week after week for the next fifty years:

- Monday—total body/plyometric training (3 hours)
- Tuesday—deadlift training (3 hours)
- Wednesday—crossfit training (3 hours)
- Thursday—15 mile run
- Friday—Pilates (1.5 hours)
- Saturday—50 miles cycling
- Sunday—abs and core (1 hour)

Oh, and I forget to tell you that he had done this routine for more than one year, and he never had taken a day off. In addition, he was the CEO of his company. He was also married with three kids!

It's possible to complete his workout routine, but is it supportable for the long run? Probably not. Even the best athletes in the world have their rest days, and they understand that those recovery days are just as important as the workout days. People who exercise without a trainer often fall into the "over workout" trap and get injured. I know this well, because I too have been there. Besides the stress and burnout we talked about in the last section, over working out is also a part of Quadrant 3: Energy Poor, Exhaustion.

Quadrant 1	Quadrant 2
Energy Rich Energy Lasting	Energy Rich Energy Non-Lastiing
Quadrant 3	Quadrant 4
Energy Poor Exhaustion	Energy Poor Lethargic

Everything in life requires a balance. When we over work out and our muscles don't get a chance to recover, they become sore. If we continually ignore the lactic acid buildup in our bodies and continue to push ourselves, we end up tearing muscles and ligaments. When we get injured, we're out of commission from working out for at least three to six months.

- Even if we can't keep up such a hefty exercise regimen, is there something we *can* do to get our energy to a high level?
- Is there an exercise that is more gentle and manageable for our bodies?
- Is there something we can do as we age that will be sustainable for the long run?
- How about one that is great for our immune systems and helps us to reduce stress in our lives?

The answer is "yes" to all of the above questions!

CHAPTER 10

Qigong – The 2,000-year-old Ancient Secret Chinese Energy Practice

"Energy is not the only basis of existence. It is the fuel that makes everything in our lives real and possible."

— Tony Robbins

In this section, I am going to teach you an ancient energy exercise that dates back more than two thousand years—from my ancestors in China—to help you manage your energy and mood. These energy exercises help you stay on top of your game and get you into the Quadrant 1: Energy Rich, Energy Lasting state.

Quadrant 1 Energy Rich Energy Lasting	Quadrant 2 Energy Rich Energy Non-Lastiing
Quadrant 3 Energy Poor Exhaustion	Quadrant 4 Energy Poor Lethargic

This is where you use the energy rich state you have created in Section I—Jump Start Your Own Energy Naturally and help make your energy longer lasting. We call this ancient energy practice *qigong* or *energy practice/energy mastery*.

Dr. Oz says, "The ancient Chinese technique of qigong is a great way tap into our natural energy and, in turn, combat the aging process." Although the *qigong* movements are simple, they open up the floodgates of energy in our bodies. The specific qigong practice we cover in this book is called lymphasizing. I have learned many different styles of qigong—in Taiwan and China for many years—but it wasn't until I studied this two-thousand-year-old lymphasizing practice that I could feel more of my internal energy during and after each practice.

Before we go into the practice, let's talk about why lymphasizing is so important to our health and energy. Remember in Section I, we learned about Nobel Prize winner Dr. Alexis Carrel who was able to keep chicken cells alive for more than twenty-seven years, as long as the cells had—do you remember which three things? If you don't remember, don't worry. We'll recap. Healthy cells need: oxygen, protection of the cell lining from physical tearing, and maintenance of their electrical fields to keep them alive forever. Lymphasizing will help us obtain all three of those things.

Let's quickly cover why we need to pay close attention to our lymph system. Our lymph system, which is like the garbage collector for our system, is the most important part of our immune system. The lymph's primary job is to clean and feed cells. When we rid our bodies of waste and provide good nutrients to our blood, our energy goes up. Surprise, surprise! It's a no brainer, right?

Well there is a problem. We don't have a mechanism in our bodies to actively clean and feed our cells. See, our circulatory system has a pump. It's called our *heart,* and it gets our blood circulating and flowing in our body. Our lymph system, however, does not have a pump—and our lymph system has three times more fluid than our circulatory system. So how do we get our lymph fluids moving to eliminate toxins and waste and provide nutrients to our cells?

You guessed it. We practice lymphasizing exercises, by gently bouncing our body up and down. I know this might sound super simple, but we instinctively lymphasize, and we don't even know it. Let me ask you this. What ritual does Muhammad Ali do before he gets into the ring to fight with George Foreman? He bounces up and down and pulls his shoulders back, right? What ritual does Michael Phelps do before he jumps into the pool to start his race? He bounces up and down to loosen up his body, right?

What ritual does Tony Robbins do before he gets on stage to deliver life transformation strategies to 135,000 attendees at an event like "Dreamforce" with Marc Benioff? He jumps on a rebounder and bounces up and down. If you never been to a Tony Robbins live seminar, the event starts at 9 a.m. and ends at 12 a.m.—sometimes going longer—for four to seven days straight. How does Tony get massive energy to deliver on stage, hour after hour, without a lot of sleep and food? He *lymphasizes*.

Remember back in Section I, I talked about my thirteen days of business travel when I stayed at the AirBNB place in Los Angeles with the two Imax stereo snorers? Let me share with you the rest of the crazy journey.

After I finished talking to the TV news producers and got booked on ten shows across the country, I went to Los Angeles International Airport the next morning to kick off the second part of the trip. I'd been invited as a senior leader for a Tony Robbins' "Date with Destiny" live seminar. I not only had to be on top of my game, I was also there to serve others—helping them overcome the challenges in their lives for the next nine days.

While at LAX waiting to get on a flight to Boca Raton in Florida, I sat in one of the thin, black leather seats, pulled out my Mac Book Air, and started working on the sections of this book. Have you ever been in the flow zone—where you are in your own world and have no idea where the time went? I mean you are so in depth with what you are doing and time seems not to matter? Yeah, that was me, typing away smiling, because I was in the *flow zone.*

Unfortunately, it doesn't work too well when we lose track of time at an airport. After finishing typing away my thoughts, I looked up at the top right of my laptop to see 10:32 a.m. "Wait a minute. Isn't my flight at 10:30?" I mumbled to myself.

I closed my laptop, packed everything up, and ran to the gate to see that the plane I was supposed to be on had just pulled away from the Jetway. The worst part was, I was going to miss the only connecting plane for the day from Atlanta, Georgia, to Boca Raton.

I ended up sleeping that night at Kansas City on an airport lounge chair where the TSA warning announcement repeated on loudspeaker every ten minutes. "So much for getting a good night's rest in a nice comfortable bed at the Boca Raton Hilton," I said to myself as I tried to get some shuteye.

Remember that I mentioned how Tony runs his seminar for fourteen hours or more per day? Yup, I was really concerned with how I was going to serve at my highest level without much sleep for the next nine days.

Whenever I felt tired or exhausted at the seminar, I would gently bounce up and down and do the qigong lymphasizing exercise. The event went underway, and everything seemed to go well until Tony asked towards the middle of the seminar, "Who here has suicidal thoughts or wants to commit suicide?"

Guess how many people stood up in my team of sixty-eight people. There were two in our group who wanted to kill themselves.

Tony can't work individually with everybody, because he only has so much time at the event. So it is part of our responsibilities as senior leaders to step up and help the attendees in our team find their own breakthroughs.

Due to client confidentiality, I am not able to disclose my interventions with the two amazing people who wanted to commit suicide, but let me ask you this to see why it's so important to be in the energy rich state and how this relates to the business world:

- Would you be able to influence someone if you ran out of patience?
- Would you be able to lead a team of high performers if you yourself were having a nervous breakdown?
- Could you tell your kids what to do when you are panicking yourself? No, of course not!

Whether you are leading a team or are a parent or are influencing someone, you need to be centered, rooted, and resourceful, don't you? As a high performer, you need to be calm in the center of the storm.

Can you imagine if there were a fire in a movie theater, and the fireman came in and started panicking—and didn't know what to do? What if you were working with a higher-level executive or someone in management who flipped out and broke down during the middle of a crisis? It would not be very confidence inspiring, would it?

In order to be centered and rooted, we need to be in the *energy rich state*, don't we?

Before helping the two suicidal attendees one by one, I took a deep breath and lymphasized to make sure I was rooted and serving them with my heart with unconditional love. I am truly happy to say that I was able to help the two of them find peace in their hearts, not because I'm so *great,* but I'm really *grateful* to have served them and helped them find their own strength through challenging times.

As high performers, often we have to stand up and serve something higher than ourselves. There is a higher purpose. Where others are not willing to go the extra mile because they are tired, we step up. We stand up and deliver, don't we? That makes us the best at what we do. That makes us a leader in our industry.

How can we use qigong in our busy, scheduled lives?

The best part of qigong is that you can do it right before an important management meeting or when you are delivering a presentation to your clients—to boost your energy. You can even wear business clothes while lymphasizing, and you don't need to worry about wrinkling them. You can also do it at the airport or hotel when you're traveling. I bounce up and down to boost my energy, presence, and "aliveness" before I come on camera at TV news stations across the country to talk about "The Three Alternatives to Cola, Coffee, and Nicotine." The morning news anchors always comment about how they love my high energy level—and how much fun they have with my TV segment.

Let's go into depth about why we feel more open after doing qigong and why Dr. Oz says this gentle practice is really great for our bodies. Although we are doing simple movements and are not pumping 80 pound barbells at the gym or sweating our butts off at 104 degrees at a Bikram Yoga class, we are still getting a workout. It just has a totally different focus.

So why is qigong so great for our optimal health? Let's imagine for a moment that our circulatory systems and lymph systems are networks of canals and floodgates that allow blood and lymph fluids to flow throughout our bodies. What happens when the canals get backed up with garbage and our floodgates can't operate properly? The flow of water stops, and those sections that are blocked keep collecting more garbage, right?

Let me ask you this: what does a pool of dirty, stillwater foster? Dirty water attracts disease carrying mosquitoes that infect us with malaria, right? It's the same with our bodies. When we have blockages and stagnation in our bodies, we put our bodies in the right environment to foster diseases such as cancer, heart disease, and arthritis. And what percentage of our bodies are comprised of water? More than 80 percent, yes?

When we open up our meridians and get our fluid moving again, we get rid of stagnation and cleanse our blood and lymph—and the positive side effect is that we have more energy that helps us look vibrant and younger.

*Key notes:

- Ideally you want to do the following exercises in the morning to help you boost your energy for the day—or before any important meeting or presentation.
- Avoid doing this sequence within three hours before you sleep.

ACTION STEP EXERCISES

Managing Your Energy for Life Exercises
(refer to Energy Rich Workbook):

Exercise a: Lymphasizing, Boosting Your Immunity, Vitality, and Energy
Exercise b: Unwinding to Allow Your Energy to Flow
Exercise c: Boosting Your Energy Meridian

Ready to experience this two-thousand-year-old ancient energy practice called qigong?

Go to your *Energy Rich Workbook* and look under Secret Energy Hack Section III – Manage Your Energy for Life.

FOMO – fear of missing out? That's what going to happen if you haven't already download the *Energy Rich Workbook* because I'll be covering a 2,000 years old ancient energy practice that Dr. Oz said, "If you want to live to 100, do Qigong everyday"?

Go to **www.AllanTing.com/IEMBookBonuses** if you haven't DOWNLOAD the FREE workbook yet.

Head towards the *Energy Rich Workbook* and look under Secret Energy Hack Section III — Manage Your Energy for Life.

CHAPTER 11

Top 7 Natural Foods to Sustain Your Quadrant 1, Energy Rich Energy Lasting State

"The greatest wealth is health."

— Virgil

a. Omega 3 and Omega 6, the Essential Oils

Most of us are oil deficient, because we have been hugely misinformed by health experts in the 1980s regarding weight loss trends. In return, oils and fats have been labeled as a public enemy—when the truth shows quite the opposite. We need essential fatty acids, called EFAs, to survive. Our bodies don't naturally produce omega 3s and 6s—both unsaturated fats—so we need to get them from foods. Other fats like omega 7 and omega 9 are saturated fats, and our body can produce them from sugar and starches. But EFAs provide many benefits to our bodies which include:

- Increased energy, stamina, and performance to help us build and repair muscles.
- Strengthening of our immune systems and control over immune and inflammatory responses in our body.
- Boost to promote great skin tone, hair, and nails, because one of the signs and symptom of EFA deficiency is brittle nails, dry and flaky skin, and dry hair.
- Reduced risk for cardiovascular disease, by lowering high levels of blood pressure and triglycerides.
- Improved brain activity, because 50 percent of our brains are comprised of fat. This boosts our memory, our vision, and how we feel throughout the day.
- A boost in weight loss by suppressing our appetite.
- Improved digestion and help with fighting leaky gut.
- Faster recovery and healing of cells and cell growth.
- Stronger bones, by helping the transport of minerals to keep bones and teeth strong.
- Boost in liver, kidney, thyroid, and adrenal gland function—and increase in beneficial male and female hormones.
- Relief of PMS.
- Enhanced and healthy child development, since a growing baby takes EFA from the pregnant mother for its nervous system development. The mother also needs EFA to replenish itself during and after pregnancy.

Now that you know how essential oils benefit your body in so many ways, let's talk about the two main challenges related to omega 3 and 6 oils.

1. The first challenge lies in getting the cleanest source of oil. We can get omega 3 from fish such as salmon, but most salmon in the US is farm grown and has one of the

highest levels of PCBs (toxic, man-made chemicals that cause cancers).

2. The second challenge is having the right ratio of omegas 3 and 6 for optimum health. Although omega 6 has increased in our food since 1850, omega 3 intake has rapidly decreased. We need both to maintain healthy cells and help fight degenerative diseases.

One of the best products I've found out there for addressing these concerns is Udo's Oil 3-6-9 Blend, and you can find it at most organic supermarkets. Note that I don't get any form of compensation from the company or founder. I recommend it, and I use the oil on a regular basis to boost my health and energy. I usually put a tablespoon of Udo's Oil in my organic steel cut oatmeal in the morning, mix it in my protein shake, or add it to my dinner soup. I admit that when I first started consuming the oil, it tasted a bit nutty, because the oil comes from organic plants. To get accustomed to the taste, start with half a teaspoon, and gradually increase the dosage.

b. Kale, The Queen of Superfood

Kale is not only low in calories with no fat, but the high fiber plant is also great for digestion. It is a powerhouse of nutrients, vitamins, and magnesium that is:

- High in iron. In fact, kale has more iron per calorie than beef. Our body needs iron for healthy cells, formation of enzymes and hemoglobin, great liver function, oxygen transport, and more.
- High in antioxidants (carotenoids and flavonoids) to help fight against cancers.

- High in calcium and vitamin C. Kale has more calcium than milk, which helps prevent aging, bone loss, and osteoporosis.
- Rich in vitamin A, which makes it great for skin and vision.
- Great for our cardiovascular system, as it helps reduce cholesterol.

Eating kale can be a bit rough due to its texture, so it's easier to palate if you blend it in a smoothie or protein shake. If you're going to eat it as a salad, I recommend marinating the leaves with lemon juice and Udo's Oil in a bowl, massage the leaves, and let it sit overnight in the refrigerator. The citric acid and rubbing helps break down the kale toughness and reduce some of the bitter taste. Then add it to the rest of the ingredients you want to include when you're ready to eat.

Here Is a Great Energy Boosting Kale Salad Recipe

- 1 bunch of kale
- Sea salt
- 1 avocado, pitted and sliced into small chunks
- 1 large carrot, shredded with a vegetable peeler
- 1 beet, sliced
- 1 small red bell pepper, deseeded and chopped
- 1 cup edamame
- 1 cup cilantro
- 1 cup Thai basil
- 2 teaspoon lime juice
- ½ cup goji berries

Ginger Vinaigrette Dressing

- ¼ cup Udo's Oil
- 2 tablespoons rice vinegar
- 1 tablespoon low sodium soy sauce or low sodium tamari
- 1 tablespoon fine grated ginger
- 3 garlic cloves, minced

Remove kale leaves from the stems, and put the leaves into a mixing bowl. Add Udo's Oil and lime juice, and massage leaves thoroughly. Leave the mixture in the refrigerator overnight. Mix in the rest of ingredients and dressing when ready to eat.

c. Goji Berries, The Secret to the Fountain of Youth

Goji has been used in Chinese medicine for thousands of years to boost vitality. My mom put goji berries in our soup on a regular basis to boost our immune systems, especially during winter. *The Journal of Alternative and Complementary Medicine* published an article in May 2008 about the positive effects of consuming goji berries. It reported improved energy levels, lower fatigue, lower stress, and improved digestion for those who consumed the berries. Even Madonna and Miranda Kerr swear by them. Other purported health benefits include:

- Beta-carotene that promotes healthy skin
- Vitamins C and E to boost your immune system and protect your vision
- Assistance in nourishing your liver and kidneys
- Antioxidants with oxygen radical absorbance capacity value
- Improved mood and well-being.

You can eat goji berries dry like trail mix or blend them in smoothies or shakes—or even add them to soups. You can also add them to kale salad. If you take blood thinners or medication for diabetes or blood pressure, do not eat goji berries, as they could react with some Western medicines. Check with your doctor first.

d. Ginger, the All Purpose Medicine Chest

Ginger has been widely used in Chinese medicine and Ayurveda (traditional Hindu medicine) through thousands of years, because of its digestive benefits. As I have mentioned, Chinese medicine treats all illness starting from digestion first—99 percent of the time—because when we get rid of toxins in our stomach and intestines, our bodies have the strength and energy to fight off other diseases. Since ginger helps boost our digestive system and offers many other health benefits, it's very prevalent in Asian food and teas. *Hawaii Medical Journal* published an article on ginger calling it "An Ancient Remedy and Modern Miracle Drug," because ginger can help:

- Fight colds and the flu.
- Improve blood circulation, since it contains chromium, magnesium, and zinc; it also helps prevent fever and chills.
- Reduce pain and inflammation.
- Improve absorption by stimulating digestive enzymes.
- Fight stomachaches.
- Reduce motion sickness and morning sickness.
- Strengthen your immune system.
- Fight coughing by opening up your lungs and helping to break down phlegm and mucus.

Grind the ginger into pulp and add 1/8 of a teaspoon into your smoothie or shake. Once you get used to the taste, add more ginger pulp into your shake or smoothie. You can also boil water with ginger slices to help you fight the flu, or throw some into your soup to boost your digestion.

e. Coconut, Coo Coo for Coconuts

The first time I went to Fiji, I had a chance to visit a local coconut facility that exports drupe all over the world. The manager gave us a tour and explained what they did to the coconuts—and all of their benefits. Women in Fiji rub their skin and wash their hair with coconut oil. No wonder they have this glowing complexion about them! It's not until recent years that we have seen the popularity of coconut water grow at places like Whole Foods and Costco warehouses, so let's talk about the multi benefits of coconut.

Coconut Water. Researchers from the American Chemical Society reported in 2012 that coconut water has five times more potassium than most sports drinks. Coconut water is a good choice for anyone who has an active lifestyle, to help replenish potassium. Plain coconut contains 61 milligrams of potassium per ounce versus most sports drinks which only have 3.75 milligrams of potassium per ounce. While most Americans don't eat enough vegetables and fruit, coconut is a great way to get potassium.

Although coconut water can help you get the right balance of electrolytes to replenish your energy, lower your blood pressure, and help build lean muscles, not all bottled coconut waters are created equal. So read the labels to make sure that there are no added sugars—and choose plain, unflavored coconut juice.

The best times to drink coconut are in the morning to get extra energy, after a long day or night working to renew your body, or after working out to replenish your electrolytes. In addition, if you sweat profusely from a workout, add a little bit of organic sea salt in your coconut water to help you retain more water.

Coconut Oil. As I mentioned earlier about the fat free diets of the eighties where all fats were all bad, many nutritionists thought coconut oil was unhealthy and contributed to heart disease. After years of research, we now know that isn't true, and coconut oil can be re-classified as a "superfood" that keeps our bodies running.

Research shows that coconut oil has many health benefits. It can help you fight off viruses and bacteria that cause illnesses. Coconut oil can help you regulate your thyroid and blood sugar, which helps improve insulin use within your body. It also improves your thyroid function to help increase energy and endurance.

Coconut oil is also a great source of lauric acid, a type of Medium Chain Triglyceride (MCT), and metabolizes differently than saturated fats from animals or cheese. Lauric acid boosts good HDL cholesterol to help you improve your overall cholesterol level. Because MCT are fatty acids of medium length, the fat goes directly to the liver after consumption.

On DoctorOz.com, Pina LoGiudice ND, LAc, co-medical director of Inner Source Health in New York, recommends organic coconut oil for all ages for skin and hair. It's a great moisturizer, because the oil contains a high amount of vitamin E.

Consuming coconut oil is simple. You can add it to your oatmeal or shake. You can bake it in your food or sauté it with vegetables. Since coconut oil has a high heat tolerance and does not go rancid and acidic like olive oil, you can use it for most cooking.

f. Wheatgrass, The One You Don't Smoke

A shot of this green juice packs a punch to your overall health. Because wheatgrass contains up to 70 percent chlorophyll, it helps build blood in your body. In fact, wheatgrass is one molecule from our hemoglobin, which is the chemical in red blood cells that carries oxygen. It helps increase the production of blood. Studies have shown that red blood cell count levels increased and blood oxygen raised dramatically when people drank wheatgrass on a consistent basis, because of chlorophyll which also helps deliver more oxygen.

This marker is a key indicator of health recovery for abnormalities, ailments, and disease. Oxygen is vital to many body processes, especially for the brain which uses 25 percent of the body's oxygen supply. High oxygen levels help support a healthy body.

Here are the other amazing benefits of wheatgrass:

- Used to detox heavy metals and drug deposits out of your body by getting rid of toxins in your liver.
- Treats cancers in alternative treatment programs.
- Helps with diabetes by improving blood sugar.
- Helps fight against bacteria with chlorophyll.
- Improves arthritis.
- Reduces high blood pressure and enhances capillaries as chlorophyll increases the function of the heart, vascular system, intestines, uterus, and lungs.
- Slows down the aging process, since chlorophyll contains superoxide dismutase and enzymes found in mature red blood cells.

Just a couple of ounces of a wheatgrass drink is equivalent to five pounds of the best vegetables. It is higher in vitamin C than an orange and has more vitamin A than a carrot. It also includes vitamin B, calcium, phosphorus, magnesium, sodium, potassium, and amino acids.

One of the best ways to drink wheatgrass is to down it like a shot, because of its taste. It does take a bit of getting used to.

Ideally, you first will want to swish it around in your mouth a few times to begin absorbing all of the chlorophyll. Note: if you have never tried wheatgrass before, you might want to have a slice of orange as a chaser handy after you drink the juice. Wheatgrass is an acquired taste!

g. Avocado, The All-Star Nutrient

"I'm staying away from avocado, because it's fattening, and I'm trying to lose weight," said a good friend of mine while we were eating Mexican food for lunch. Going back to the eighties' zero fat diets, avocado fell into the "bad food" group due to the fact that 85 percent of its calories come from fat. Although it is a high-fat food, research has shown that this powerhouse fruit offers many health benefits:

- **Better nutrient intake and diet quality,** because avocado helps lower LDL (bad cholesterol), according to the *Archives of Medical Research*. The journal published an article stating that an "avocado enriched diet can improve lipid profile in healthy and especially in mild hypercholesterolemic patients, even if hypertriglyceridemia (combined hyperlipidemia) is present." The research found that patients who ate a good amount of avocado experienced a 22 percent decrease in triglyceride levels and LDL—and an 11 percent increase in HDL (good cholesterol). What's a good amount of avocado to eat? That depends on your lifestyle, activities, weight, and metabolic rate. Remember, moderation is key. Eat balanced meals. Half of an avocado is about one-third of your normal fat intake.

- **Weight management.** People who regularly eat avocado help lower their body weight and BMI (Body Mass Index) and enjoy a slimmer waistline. *The Nutrition Journal* published a study showing a correlation between eating avocados and metabolic syndrome—a group of risk factors that includes coronary artery disease, stroke, and diabetes.
- **Cancer fighting properties.** A team of scientists found that "individual and combinations of phytochemicals from the avocado fruit may offer an advantageous dietary strategy in cancer prevention." When you eat one cup of fresh avocado with a salad of mixed spring leaves, carrots, and spinach, it boosts the absorption of carotenoid by 200 percent to 400 percent because of oleic acid. Oleic acid is a monounsaturated fatty acid that helps your digestion build transport molecules (chylomicrons) and carry carotenoids antioxidants, one of the key roles to cancer prevention.
- **Arthritis fighting capabilities from its phytosterols—** that includes beta-sitosterol, campesterol, and stigmasterol. They are the key ingredients to keep our inflammatory systems in control. Many researchers have shown that consuming avocados for arthritis—both osteoarthritis and rheumatoid arthritis—helps reduce and alleviate pain.

Avocado Smoothie

Other than eating avocado in a salad, I love avocado smoothies. Here is one of my favorite smoothies recipes:

- 1 avocado
- 2-1/2 cups soaked almonds
- 8 cups water
- 1-1/2 cups dates

SECTION III

Game Changer Questions

"You see, in life, lots of people know what to do, but few people actually do what they know. Knowing is not enough! You must take action."

— Tony Robbins

1. If you're going to experience even more of the flow zone, you would have to...
2. How would being in the flow zone affect your life? Even if you had 10 percent more energy, how would it help you—at work? With your Income? Back at home? How about your overall wellness?
3. If you were to take better care of yourself, physically and mentally, what would be the three things you would start doing to manage your energy for life?

Advanced Energy State: The Joy of Pure Energy

The Gin and Juice of Neuroscience
The Mind and Body Connection
The Science of Being Thankful and Grateful
The Emotional Detox and Cleansing Through Sound and Vibration

Secret Energy Hack Section IV Overview

"Calm mind brings inner strength and self-confidence, so that's very important for good health."

— Dalai Lama

The Top CEOs of America and Congressman Are Coming Out of the Closet

A year ago, I attended a conference where Arianna Huffington, co-founder of *The Huffington Post*, gave a resounding speech about work life balance. No longer is she putting her health after her career, as most Americans have been conditioned to do. She said, "I fainted, hit my head on my desk, broke my cheekbone, and had to get five stitches around my right eye. It got me thinking about what kind of life I was leading. I was getting four to five hours of sleep a night. I had to slow down and reevaluate the choices I was making."

She continued, "The toughest part was disconnecting from all my devices, especially as I was running an online media company. I thought people would need an answer, things would be left undone. I had to get better at living with incompletion. I learned to say no to things I wanted to do. The reality was I couldn't do it all."

Arianna wasn't the only one who suffered from fatigue and burnout from overworking. In 2011, Lloyds Banking Group chief António Horta-Osório was forced to take two months' leave because of extreme fatigue. *The Wall Street Journal* reported a Harvard Medical School study where 96 percent of senior leaders felt somewhat burnt out, and a third of them described it as extreme. A CEO leave of absence such as this not only affects shareholders' confidence, but also leaves the employees uncertain about the company's future—and their own struggle with burnouts. You just don't hear about any CEOs taking month-long vacations!

It only took five stitches and a broken cheekbone to wake Arianna up from overworking. But you don't have to get to the point where you are injured or ill. You can prevent burnout by being proactive.

This section includes simple and effective strategies that successful people use to avoid burnout, consistently bring their A games to work, and come back home with a full presence.

> *"Save the green mountain, you won't worry about having no firewood to burn."*
>
> — Chinese Adage

Unplug to Recharge

Because the growth of smartphones has exploded over the last five years, many Americans are working more than ever. Using a smartphone for work is really a double edged sword, because while it enhances productivity and mobility, you are also handcuffed to it. In the beginning of this book, I mentioned that *USA Today* reported that eight out of ten Americans are always working, because it's so easy to connect to the Internet via mobile devices.

In 2013, the average mobile users "watched about two hours of video per month, listened two hours of audio, made five video calls, and downloaded two apps over their cellular network," according to *Forbes*, and "by 2018, we're expected to watch twenty hours of video per month, listen to ten hours of video, make eleven video calls and download twenty apps."

ComScore reported that more Internet traffic has been logged on smartphones and tablet devices than ever before. According to their report, 60 percent of Internet usage from Feb 2013 to May 2014 happened on mobile devices. So what information do people access on the Internet? The vast majority—99.5 percent—of people access content including checking email and reading online. In addition, as of 2014, 58 percent of American adults have smartphones, 32 percent of American adults own an e-reader, and 42 percent of American adults own a tablet.

The problem with Arianna and many Americans is that we are always connected. Or to be more accurate, it's like we are tethered to our devices, to the point that our brains hardly get a chance to stop thinking.

We live in a very interesting time when we can access almost any information any time at our fingertips, thanks to Google, whereas about one hundred years ago, people like Henry Ford used to have to thumb through big catalogs of books to find similar answers. In the fast paced, twenty-first century, our brains are stimulated and bombarded with information now more than ever, and it's only going to get worse. Let me ask you:

- Have you ever felt a phantom vibration of your phone—wherein you pick up your smartphone, thinking it vibrated, even if it didn't ring or vibrate?

- Do you have an itch, an addiction, to check your mobile phone when you're waiting for your coffee at the Starbucks line?
- Do you sleep next to your phone at night, because you want to make sure you didn't miss any calls, text messages, or other updates?
- Can you imagine what your life would be like without your cell phone?

Yes, I get it if you are struggling to think about breaking free, because life would be really hard for me without my iPhone. I use it to take selfies on Instagram, listen to the latest songs from Maroon 5 on iTunes, check email, search the Internet, check stock and weather reports, and connect to Google Maps.

Our smartphones are incredibly useful. However, we need to kick the bad addiction of needing a 24/7 relationship with the Internet. I'm not saying to break up your relationship with the Internet altogether. Just agree to take a mental vacation from time to time. I made a habit of not checking my iPhone after 9 p.m., and I usually turn my iPhone off for one weekend every ninety days, so that I can spend some quality time with my friends and family. Unplugging can help your mind detox and relax. Would you ever not empty your garbage can underneath the kitchen sink? Of course not! Just like we need to get rid of the leftover organic vegan tofu pizza left in the trash, we also need to empty our mental trash bin as well.

Can't Sleep? Join the "Dark Side," Young Skywalker

In the beginning of this section, we talked about how the Center for Disease Control reported that "Insufficient Sleep Is a Public Health Epidemic," stating that an estimated fifty million to seventy million American adults chronically experience sleep disorders and insomnia.

One of the biggest culprits of sleep disorders is accessing our smartphones, tablets, or flat screen TVs before we sleep, because of the blue light they emit. The blue wavelength is great during the day, because it helps us boost attention and brighten our mood. However, when we receive blue lights at night, they disrupt our circadian rhythms—or our biological clocks that regulate when we wake up and when we sleep.

Although all types of light can suppress melatonin, the hormone that helps you control wake and sleep cycles, the blue wavelength does it more powerfully. Harvard Medical School did a research study wherein participants received 6.5 hours of blue light exposure to green light of comparable brightness. The powerful blue wave suppressed melatonin almost twice as long as the green light. The blue light also shifted the circadian rhythms twice as much.

When I was on ABC News talking about how to boost energy naturally, one of the main anchors asked me what to do when we can't sleep at night, because she also suffers from low energy. Before I gave her the remedy, the first thing I asked her was, "You must use your smartphone at night before you sleep, don't you?"

She said, "How do you know?"

And I asked her, "When you finally fall asleep, your brain is probably still doing mental somersaults and calisthenics, isn't it?"

She said, "You're right again and I got to stop playing Candy Crush before bed!"

When we use devices that emit blue lights, our biological clocks still think it's daytime. This throws our circadian rhythms out of whack. So stay away from surfing on Amazon, eBay, or WalMart. com two to three hours before you sleep. The alternative is to wear blue light blocking glasses if you still need to scratch your itch.

And if you don't think this matters, know that WebMD published an article October 5, 2010, showing that sleep disorders may cause headaches, obesity, diabetes, heart disease, depression, and even early death. Do you still think sleep is not that important?

Who Are The New Business Elite?

Do you ever wonder how the iconic Steve Jobs got his creativity? How did he bring Apple stocks from $0.45 in 1998 to $1.16 in 2014? If you had bought Apple with just $100 at $0.45 a share and sold it in 2014, you would have made more than $11,000! He managed to out maneuver the titans of the industry: defeating Rio MP3 players with iPod and beating Nokia in the saturated mobile phone sector with iPhone. More importantly, Steve created raving customers who would wait in lines for days before the new launch of each iPhone.

Would you want to know the ingredients to Steve's secret sauce? At Steve's funeral, he gave his friends and family his last parting gift, a copy of *Autobiography of a Yogi* in a wooden box. When Steve traveled to India, he realized that his intuition was his greatest gift. His intuition came from awakening his self-realization through a consistent practice of Zen meditation. Whereas his archrivals looked at how to copy competitors and make their own products better—and how to build their PCs faster and cheaper—Steve looked at how to revolutionize the entire industry starting with what the consumers really wanted.

In order to find out what the world really wanted, Steve looked at the world inside out through Zen meditation. More and more top CEOs, executives, and business leaders are coming out of the closet and telling people that they meditate. Marc Benioff, CEO of Salesforce, stated in a 2013 *Huffington Post* article, "I enjoy meditation, which I've been doing for over a decade—probably to help relieve the stress I was going through when I was working at Oracle. Meditation is a major part of my life," Benioff said. "It's been that way for a couple of decades, and that is something that I am in line with Steve Jobs on." Other CEOs like Mark Bertolini from Aetna, Jeff Weiner from Linkedin, Rick Rubin former Columbia Records, John Mackey from Whole Foods, Evan Williams of Twitter, Soledad O'Brien from Starfish Media (and CNN anchor) also meditate—according to the article. Even Ohio Congressman Tim Ryan meditates, and he's from the Midwest!

According to a CNBC.com article on March 19, 2013, when the CEO of Aetna, Mark Bertolini, broke his neck from a skiing accident, he took painkillers for a year. It wasn't until he started practicing yoga and meditation that he found natural pain relief. Oh, and the other major positive side effect was the benefit of making better decisions at work. He even introduced a twelve-week yoga and mindfulness program to the employees at Aetna. The participating employees experienced a dramatic decrease in stress levels and increased productivity. He stated that he wanted to roll this program out and make it available to 34,000 employees at Aetna.

"Okay great. You are telling me all these executives are meditating. How does that apply to my work and personal life?" you might ask.

Let me share with you how I went from near homeless to healing my chronic stress and fatigue—and taking my life and career to the next level. I started practicing Zen meditation more than ten years ago and felt firsthand how it alleviated my stress from work and my neck, shoulder, and back pain.

Sitting in stillness wasn't easy, as my mind raced through thoughts like, "Oh crap, I've got to respond back to that email," or "I'm getting hungry, and that sun dried tomato basil pesto pasta sounds great right now," or "This is the longest five minutes in stillness ever!" The endless chatter kept flowing in my mind, and I just couldn't stay focused on meditation.

If you have meditated before, you know what I'm talking about. If you have not meditated before, this would be a precursor to the challenges you are going to face.

But through consistent practice, my mind started to slow down and unwind from thoughts, and one day, magic happened. I was working on a $500,000 request for proposal (RFP) for a municipal power company in the Midwest. My team and I had about thirty days to finish the proposal, and my section of the proposal was done in a week. I had tasked one of the sales engineers to work on the technical portion of the proposal, and he dragged his feet. Every Monday, I would check with him on the proposal status, and he would say, "Yeah yeah, I'm working on it," even though he was busy with other tasks.

It wasn't until T minus one day that this sales engineer pushed the panic button and said, *"Houston, we have a problem."* He realized that he had to talk to the vice president of research and development to help answer the questions in the RFP. The government takes the RFP timeline very seriously! If you deliver even one minute late to their door, you will not be considered in the selection process— even if you have the best mousetrap in the world.

By the time my sales engineer and I had finally finished the RFP, it was 9:30 p.m., and we had missed the FedEx overnight shipping deadline. I even called around to other couriers, but again, we had missed the deadline.

Prior to meditation, I would have focused on the problem and thrown a huge tantrum at my sales engineer for dragging his feet. Yelling and being angry with him wouldn't have solved our problem at hand. Thoughts of choking him did cross my mind though, but again, that was not going to help solve the problem.

Instead, I said, "Okay, this is a challenge. There must be a way we can get this $500,000 RFP delivered to Tennessee. I am not going down without a fight. I worked too hard on this." So I took a deep breath, put aside how much I wanted to strangle my colleague, and changed my focus. I told him to go home, since there was nothing else he could have done at that time. Immediately, I called my manager.

I told her, "Look, we missed the cutoff time, but there is still a chance for us to deliver this proposal in time. I will hand deliver the proposal. I checked the airfare from San Francisco to Chattanooga. It's about $1,000—totally worth spending for a $500,000 proposal."

My manager said, "Let me check with our VP, and I will call you back."

Ten minutes later, she called and said, "VP said no go on the travel. I'm sorry."

By this time, it was 2 a.m., and I started packing my bag to head home—feeling defeated and disgusted at the situation. I had come up with something totally out of the box, and my idea was shut down cold. *A $500,000 proposal,* I thought. It would have been one of the biggest government opportunities for the software company.

Again, I took a deep breath, meditated for five minutes to clear anger and frustration out of my head, and said, "Roll with the punches. Tomorrow is another day," like Dicky Fox said in *Jerry McGuire,* and I left the office.

I drove home on the empty street of 19th Avenue—one of the busiest streets in San Francisco—at 2:30 a.m. As I cruised along listening to meditation music, a question randomly popped into my head. I thought to myself, *I know Kinkos is opened 24/7, but can they meet all of my printing and delivery needs?*

Since this was pre smartphone days, when I didn't have Internet access at my fingertips, I had to go home and fire up my Pentium II desktop computer. I got on the Internet and looked for Kinkos in Chattanooga and immediately gave them a call.

A man with a Southern drawl answered the phone, "Hello, this is Kinkos. May I help you?"

I said, "I know you guys do print jobs, but can you receive files and print? Would you be able to burn those files on CDs? Would you be able to deliver to a local client?"

"Sure, we can. We can do it all." the young man said.

I quickly turned around and headed back into the office, got on my PC at work, and sent off the files. Then I called a local 24/7 pizzeria for a delivery. I know pizza is not a part of the high performance diet, but after all, I am human—and it's okay to deviate off the track once in a blue moon!

Anyhow, as I was scarfing down the pepperoni pizza at 5:30 a.m., I received a call from Kinkos. The rep said, "Sir, your proposal has been done. We'll give you a call when it's delivered."

I called my manager and told her how I had overcame the delivery problem, and that it had only cost $184, including the medium pepperoni pizza.

She was thrilled and said, "Oh my gosh, Allan, you're a genius! Why didn't I think of that?"

At 1:45 p.m., Kinkos gave me a call and said my package was delivered before the 3:15 p.m. deadline. I was more than thrilled that I had pulled this off. I felt that it happened because I used meditation as an instrument to:

1. Clear my head, and
2. Redirect my attention from focusing on the problem to focusing on the solution.

Unfortunately, I wasn't around long enough to see if the RFP that I had submitted had won, because I was recruited to another company. However, I used the same exact meditation and focus at the new high tech software company and achieved the ranking of number one account manager of the year in 2006; I surpassed more than 180 percent of my quota.

If you are looking for more clarity, more creativity, and more focus at work, then meditation is one of the best methods—hands down.

Are you still wondering if meditation is good for you? You know that Oprah meditates too, right? If Oprah meditates, then it must be great! Joking aside, let's discuss the science of meditation.

CHAPTER 12

The Gin and Juice of Neuroscience Alchemy: SIP (Somatosensory, Insula, Prefrontal Cortex)

*"Every thought is a seed. If you plant crab apples,
don't count on harvesting golden delicious."*

— Bill Meyer

Still don't want to drink the meditation Kool-Aid? Here is what science have to say. Most of the time, we go through life without awareness of our minds or thoughts. Yet the mind/brain is like a supercomputer on steroids that is capable of solving complex problems, experiencing all levels of emotions, and much, much more. Unlike a computer that comes with user guides and training manuals, no one ever gives us a set of manuals on how our brain works when we are born.

So how do we train our minds, our own super duper computers, to have better attention, more focus, more happiness, more passion, and a greater ability to feel more energetic and alive?

Scientists may have started to unlock the keys on the neuroscience of mediation. In fact, meditation studies have exploded exponentially since 1990. In 2005, Sara Lazar, a research scientist at Harvard Medical School's Massachusetts General Hospital presented her findings on meditation comparing cortical thickness in people who mediated and those who had not. What they found was experienced meditators had an increased thickness in insula, prefrontal cortex, and somatosensory cortex.

An increase in thickness? Does that mean we become even more stubborn and thick headed when we meditate? Not quite. Let's talk about how these parts of the brain govern our everyday lives.

Somatosensory: What's the Somato With You Today?

The somatosensory cortex is our body's complex sensory system that gives us the ability to feel heat when we touch the hot burning stove with our hands—or feel the cold snow with our feet when we walk outside barefoot during the winter in Alaska. These receptors cover both the motor areas of our body—such as eyes, neck, thumbs, and feet—and the sensory areas of our body—like tongue, fingers, toes, etc. This cortex also is responsible for the pain we feel in our bodies—both acute pain, like feeling our feet throbbing when a cylinder block falls on our toes, and chronic pain, like having a dull ache in our backs. What is worse is that if you've ever experienced chronic pain, it feels like you're trapped with it, and you have no way out.

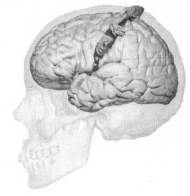

So does meditation help ease the pain? Is there a key to unlock this pain cage so that we can go on with our lives?

Researchers from Wake Forest University did an interesting study where they purposely induced pain into their human test subjects who never had meditated before. They used a heating device on a small area of the participants' skin to heat it to 120 degrees Fahrenheit (most people would find this painful) and hold it for five minutes. Don't ask me how they bribed their participants to take part in getting burned, but the researchers did, and they used MRI technology to measure the subjects' brains before and after meditation training.

With only four twenty-minute meditation classes, "Every participants' pain rating level were reduced, with decreases ranging from 11 to 93 percent," Zeidan said. In addition, the scan showed that meditation vastly reduced primary somatosensory cortex activities, which are largely responsible for feeling how intense the pain stimulus is. Prior to meditation, the activity in the somatosensory region was very high. On the flip side, the scan was not able to detect the pain-processing area when participants meditated through the scans.

Even the military is looking into meditation to help veterans cope with Post Traumatic Stress Disorder (PTSD) when they come back from tours of duty in Iraq and/or Afghanistan. Currently one in five veterans has PTSD, and returning vets with PTSD have very high suicide rates. For several years, researchers from Stanford have been studying how breath-based meditation has helped soldiers with their traumatic events of flashbacks, nightmares, and major anxiety.

Whereas the traditional treatment of therapy and medication are not always effective, "Overall, the results were fruitful. It resulted in reduced PTSD symptoms, anxiety, and respiration rate," Emma Seppala, associate director of Stanford Center for Compassion and Altruism Research and Education, said.

"So how do I get started?" you might be wondering. I will teach you a step-by-step meditation guide shortly at the end of this section.

The good news is, meditation is easy to start. The bad news is, it's not easy to calm our minds down. But like working out at a gym, meditation practitioners strengthen and create new connections in their brain cells over time. With consistent practice, meditation may improve insulation of neurons from getting damaged and also help enable the communication between the neurons.

"But I thought that scientists said our brains peak in adolescence and atrophy as we get older?"

In one study, Eileen Luders, PhD, an assistant professor in the Department of Neurology at the UCLA School of Medicine looked at the embodied mind by hooking up meditation practitioners with electroencephalograms (EEG) and scanning their brains with magnetic resonance imaging (MRIs) to scan their cortical activities. They were looking at how meditation changed the brain and busted a myth that scientists used to believe.

In the old world, scientists believed that our brains fully mature as adults and slowly decrease as we get age past our prime. This breakthrough in the new research is like busting the myth that "the world is flat." However, Luder found that experienced meditators in the study (five to forty-six years of meditation) had more gray matter in areas of their brains. Gray matter is responsible for holding attention and regulating emotions. And increasing gray matter is like adding more horsepower to your Intel processor in your MacBook to help you process information more effectively. As Luders says, "Today we know that everything we do, and every experience we have, actually changes the brain."

Eileen and her colleagues studied twenty-two meditators and twenty-two matching age non-meditators and found that those who practiced meditation over five years had more gray matter in their brains. Besides being important for regulating emotions and having better attention, having more gray matter also makes our brains process information more effectively. This also helps us make more mindful choices.

Let me ask you this:

- Would you like to learn the secrets of the high performance mindset?
- How would your life be more beneficial if you had more focus?
- How would it be if you were able to manage your stress level even better?
- What would you do if you had even more happiness in your life?

Are you still kind of worried about "getting it right" when it comes to meditation? As long as you give a well-intended practice, you'll have a great practice session. Remember, training your mind is like riding a bicycle. When you first start, it may be a bit challenging, but once you get the hang of it, you'll be cruising right along.

Meet Insula, Your Intuition's Best Friend

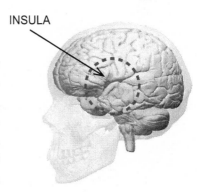

INSULA

Remember how upset I was for not being able to deliver the Request For Proposal in time, and how I spent five minutes meditating to clear my head before leaving work at 2 a.m.? Because I stayed cool, calm, and collected, my intuition regarding Kinkos kicked in. That is what the insula cortex does. It helps boost the emotional intelligence (EQ) in our everyday lives.

The insula cortex, located deep inside our cerebral cortex, plays one of the key critical roles in controlling our health and wellness. It is responsible for body sensations like self-awareness, regulating our body homeostasis, and regulating our feelings and emotions. One of the other reasons why I held myself back from throwing a tantrum at my colleague was that I exercised compassion and looked at the situation from his point of view. Perhaps the sales engineer had some personal issues he was dealing with at home, and work was not his top priority at that instant. We all have been there—where work was not a priority in our lives. Maybe our kids are sick at home with a 105 degree fever, or someone close to us passed away. Through meditation, I was able to find empathy and compassion, and my sales engineer always respected me for how I handled the situation.

Show More Prefrontal Cortex to your Wife

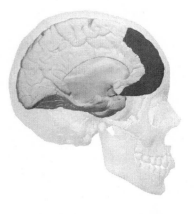

Get your mind out of the gutter. We're talking about having more presence in our lives, not flashing at your wife.

Have you ever tried multi-tasking, like flipping through your work email on your iPhone and speaking to your spouse at the same time? How did that work out for you? Did you get caught up with your own thoughts while she was speaking?

She says, "Do you like these shoes? Do they match my dress?"

You say, "Yes Honey, that dress looks great on you. Yes, uh-huh, you look great," as you're flipping through your smartphone.

Most of us experience this many times during the day as we get caught up with our thoughts. When that happens, we mentally escape into another world, and we become less present. When we're less present, we lose out on smelling the roses that are around us. In psychology, this condition is called the additional blink. The more *additional blink* that we have, the less we notice and more we miss out on life.

The prefrontal cortex part of the brain which covers the front part of the lobe is responsible for holding our attention and regulating our emotions. It's also the executive function of our brain that helps us determine what is good and bad, sort through conflicting thoughts, predict the future, and judge the situation so we can determine how it's decided.

So take a wild guess which activity can help you be more present with your wife? You guessed it. Meditation can help. Not only would you be more present with your spouse, but meditation could also help you focus better at work.

Richard Davidson, director of the Waisman Laboratory for Brain Imaging and Behavior at the School of Medicine and Public Health at the University of Wisconsin, and his research team have shown how meditation can boost your concentration in two ways. The first is that it helps you focus and cut out the white noises that are around you, literally. Second, meditation can help you notice more of what is happening around you—helping you smell the roses more often and offering you a richer respective in life.

To find out how the meditators' brain activity functioned, the scientists inserted the participants into an MRI machine and measured their brain activities during meditation, while frequently blasting the subjects with disturbing noises. Richard said:

We found that regions of the brain that are intimately involved in the control and regulation of attention, such as the prefrontal cortex, were more activated in the long-term practitioners... Most people, if they heard a baby screaming, would have some emotional response. They do hear the sound, we can detect that in the auditory cortex, but they don't have the emotional reaction.

Researchers also hooked an EEG on participants to measure the moment-by-moment electrical activities and track patterns in their brains. The result was that the meditation practitioners used less brain resources when they were asked to track multiple targets. Because they used less mental energy to see the first targets, their brains gave them more resources to pay attention to what was coming up next. It became easier for their brains to pay attention.

So the net effect is that researchers believe meditation may help us focus more by helping us take our brains back under our control. To those who feel like a chicken running around without a head, meditation just might get you *ahead* in life, at work, and in your relationship. No pun intended.

This experiment has not been thoroughly tested in labs, but I have a hunch that there is a correlation between paying more attention to your wife and getting lucky. Yes I said it, "The more you pay attention to your wife with more presence and without your mind wandering elsewhere, the happier you are in bed."

Try it for a week, and see how your sex life changes. Drop me a note. I'd love to hear how this experiment is working out for you; contact me through info@allanting.com.

ACTION STEP EXERCISES

Ready to take on the challenge of meditation?

Here is an invitation for you to head over to the *Energy Rich Workbook*. Look under Secret Energy Hack Section IV – Advanced Energy State: The Joy of Pure Energy for the clarity of mind meditation, stress and anxiety reduction meditation and blissful meditation exercises. It may seem difficult at first but if you stick with it and have some patience, it'll pay dividends and you'll see great results!

Haven't downloaded the *Energy Rich Workbook?!?* Go to **www.AllanTing.com/IEMBookBonuses** and head towards the Secret Energy Hack Section IV – Advanced Energy State: The Joy of Pure Energy.

Meditation Exercises (refer to Energy Rich Workbook):

Exercise a: Clarity of Mind Meditation
Exercise b: Stress and Anxiety Relief Meditation
Exercise c: Blissful Meditation

CHAPTER 13

Mind and Body Connection

"Your beliefs become your thoughts, Your thoughts become your words, Your words become your actions, Your actions become your habits, Your habits become your values, Your values become your destiny."

— Mahatma Gandhi

One day, a colleague of mine dropped by my desk when I was working at a very well-known software company. He stood over my cubicle, put his arms on top of the beige cubicle divider, leaned over with his 6 foot 5 inch, 265-pound frame, stared at me, and said, "Allan, Man, I hate you."

While seated, I turned around and looked at him, smiled, and said, "Say what?!?"

Again he said, "I hate you, Man," just like that, out of the blue.

I paused for a moment, again smiled, and said, "Why do you hate me?"

He looked at me with frustration and said, "Man, because you're always so happy."

I started laughing, and he became even more upset and walked away.

What he didn't know was that I had just recently separated from another four-year relationship. I was going through my own emotional roller coaster, but the reason why I still kept my cool was because I knew how to manage my energy.

If I didn't have a daily practice managing my energy, I would not have had the strength to stay focused at work. If I were emotional and bitter, I would not have had the resources or patience to understand my clients and their needs—or to manage the million dollar accounts. I was able to tap into my resources, because I had a routine practice.

Have you ever had a fight with your spouse, and your upset emotions affected your work performance? Did these fights ever spill over to other areas in your life because of your bad mood?

Take a moment to reflect on this next sentence: *"When you are angry, you are angry at the world."*

Think about the last time you were really upset at something. Even though you were upset at one person or an event, were you upset at everything that was around you?

As busy office professionals or entrepreneurs, our lives are really easy, right? I mean we work fewer than ten hours a week. We have incredibly difficult tasks to solve with really tight deadlines to meet at work. Back at home, our kids are well behaved, our spouse is always in agreement with us, and we never worry about our money and finances.

You're never stressed out, right? We re-label stress out as over achieving. We don't have time for stress!

I don't know about you, but stress is always in my life. Do you remember from Section II that stress is one of the biggest drainers of energy?

Have you ever wondered why some successful people have everything in life? They love their jobs. They are so in love. They have great intimate relationships. They have this glow about them. They are so happy that you ask, "Why are they so happy?" and it kind of pisses you off, right?

Well, these happy and successful people weren't born like this. Fundamentally, they understand that if we can control our emotions, then we can control our outlook in life. When you can control your outlook in life, you will have more focus and feel less overwhelmed and out of control. This is where the magic starts to happen, and that magic spills over to every aspect of your life—relationship, finances, career, spirituality, relationship with yourself—and you will get into what the high performers called "the flow zone."

Let's go into detail about how our minds and bodies integrate together. Traditional Chinese medicine says that different part of our organs hold different emotions. It's not until recently that science has been able to validate that theory. Let me ask you this:

- Have you ever felt nauseous before giving a public presentation?
- Did you ever get "gut-wrenching" feelings during a job interview?
- Did you ever get "butterflies" in your stomach when you were about to go for your first kiss on a date?

Physically, you felt something in your stomach, didn't you? This may seem like common sense to you, because we even use these expressions to describe how we feel for a reason. However, remember that common sense is not common knowledge.

In the book *The Second Brain*, by Michael Gershon, MD, discusses that scientists have found that our stomach linings have same molecular make-ups as our brains. In fact, scientists use to think that our brains carried information to the gut, but in reality 90 percent of the vagus nerve fibers send the information to the brain. That probably explains why we get "sick to the stomach" and feel queasy when we are under tremendous stress, rather than feeling the discomfort in our brains. This finding has opened up a new study of medicine called neurogastroenterology, as medical science has finally caught up with the "gut feel."

Actually, if we pay close attention in our everyday language pattern, we knew this all along. But we just never made the connection, and science still has a long way to catch up.

For instance, I'm sure of how you felt when you broke up with your first real love. Did you feel "heartbroken?" Remember that number one single from Toni Braxton, "Un-break My Heart"? *"Un-break my heart, say you'll love me again. Undo this hurt you caused when you walked out the door and walked out of my life."*

So what happens next when our hearts get broken? We go through this emotional roller coaster ride of resentment, anger, sadness, and soon our later we start bawling with tears, right? We literally feel pain and tightness in the thoracic part of our bodies, don't we?

The tension that we feel in our chest is from the lungs, which is the organ that holds grief and sadness. Here is another common sense but not common knowledge example. What happens to our physiology when we cry? We sniff sniff, sob sob, with very short and quick breaths, right? When we sniff sniff, we activate our lungs.

On the flip side, our lungs also hold the positive emotions of aspiration and inspiration. Have you ever had an "a-ha" moment, wherein you had a breakthrough, a moment of clarity and epiphany? Did you feel a spark inside? Did it ignite a passion in you? How did you breath afterwards? Did you take a deep inhale followed by a quick exhale? Try saying the words "a-ha" a few times, and notice your breath. Did you feel more opened up and lifted? It feels great, doesn't it?

My wife and I were on our honeymoon in Hawaii, and we met up with a good friend of ours for dinner. While we're slurping on good oxtail ramen noodles, her husband said to us that he had had one of those days when he felt uber frustrated with the people that he worked with in his real estate mortgage business.

He said, "Often times, I have no control how fast escrow closes or how and when the loan will get approved."In his job, he gets bombarded with calls and emails from the buyer's real estate agent, the seller's real estate agent, the underwriters, and the appraiser. They hound him for updates, even though he has no control over how fast the mortgage companies approve the loan or how fast escrow goes through.

I asked him, "Where do you feel it in your body when you feel like you're out of control?"

He thought for a moment and said, "My stomach."

I said, "Most people binge eat when they are under stress, even when they are not hungry."

His wife said, "Yes, he eats whenever he gets stressed out."

I asked him, "What happens after you eat? How do you feel?

He said, "I feel much better, more calm after I eat."

I asked, "Do you know why that is? Where does blood go after you eat a heavy meal? It moves from your head and towards your stomach for digestion, right? When this happens, your energy moves downwards, right?"

There are certain foods that when we eat, we feel light—leafy foods like organic kale salad and most vegetables. Then there are heavy foods like pizza, biscuits, spaghetti with meatballs, Southern fried chicken with mashed potatoes, and mac and cheese. Don't we feel more comfortable just thinking about them?

It's the thickness of the food that makes us feel like home. Hence, the term "comfort food."

When we eat under stress, we are training our brains for a quick fix. We condition our brains to associate eating more mac and cheese with feeling more calm and certain. Unfortunately, this has a negative, downward spiraling effect to our weight and our health. We don't gain twenty pounds in one day, but if we keep conditioning our brains over time, we become our own Pavlov's dog, salivating under stress. Similar to drug addiction, we binge on food, and that's how we gain fifty pounds over time. I know this well, because I've been there—as I mentioned in the beginning of this book.

Now that we have a better understanding of how our organs play a key role with our emotions, each organ has its own related emotion. When we experience a consistent emotion such as anger on a weekly basis, the angry state imbalances the liver. Over a period of time, the imbalanced liver is agitated and can produce symptoms of anger that lead to a self-perpetuating cycle.

Does that mean we should not feel any emotions and brush situations underneath the carpet and forget about them? Not exactly. When we are experiencing the full range of emotion, we are living. Even The Holiness, Dalai Lama, grieved when his brother died. It is important not to push emotions away, because those emotions will come back to haunt you later. However, it's only when we relive the same emotions over and over or with full intensity that our organs become imbalanced. Instead, allow the emotions to flow through you like a leaf flowing through a river, and don't hold on to them. Don't keep crying over spilled milk!

Does that mean we should not feel joy as well? Funny you should ask. There is an adage in Chinese, "Over joy, foster grief." Most people want to have as much joy in their lives as possible, so why would I suggest that you don't have more joy? An emotional imbalance isn't caused by happiness, rather by over stimulation or over excitement—as unexpected good news shocks our system as well. Keep in mind, there is a difference between joy and contempt versus joy and over-excitement.

Remember that funny commercial wherein an older couple is on a winter excursion, staying at a house in the middle of nowhere, and it's pouring down snow? The excited woman handcuffs herself to the bed and throws away the key, while an equally thrilled old man jumps on the bed and straddles her. During the middle of the joy and excitement, the old man gets a myocardial infarction where he holds his hands by his heart, because he is in such pain, and he collapses on top of his wife. Yes, that would be *over joy*.

I know this seems to be common sense, but again, not common knowledge, so let's do an experiment together. I'd like you to imagine a moment in your life when you were sleeping and dreamt that you were falling. This could be missing a step as you were going down a flight of stairs, and you were tumbling down, or you were climbing a ladder and you missed a step and fell—or even you were floating in the sky, and all of a sudden, the wind beneath your wing dropped, and you were falling uncontrollably.

Whatever falling dreams you've had, I'd like you to go there now and take a minute to recall the sensation back then—see what you saw, hear what you heard, and feel what you felt.

Ready? Go.

What part of your body responded when you fell? Did you feel it in your heart, like literally your heart felt like it dropped? Or did you feel a bit queasy in your stomach?

Now notice the ground underneath you, supporting you. You didn't trip. You haven't fallen yet; but you're still able to recall the sensation, and you physically feel it in your body. People feel this because when we feel fear, we feel it in our heart organ. Fear also causes anxiety, which affects our lung organ and large intestine.

Does this start to make sense?

Here is a breakdown of our organs and emotions associated to them:

Emotions	Organs	Conditions
Anger: Rage, Resentment, Frustration	Liver	• Higher blood pressure • Blurry vision • Stroke • Headaches • Asthma • Pain around the liver • Nose bleed and vessels burst because of weak spleen • Impairs decision making due to anger and inability to think straight
Grief or Sadness	Lungs	• Tightness in the chest • Excessive crying • Asthma • More prone to cold and flu • Skin problems
Worry and Anxiety	Lungs and Large Intestines	• Shortness of breath/ hyperventilation • Long term leads to ulcerative colitis that causes inflammation and sores in the digestive tract • Diarrhea and improper bowel movement or gas

Pensiveness and Over Thinking	Spleen	• Chronic fatigue • Lethargy • Inability to concentrate
Fright	Gallbladder	• Indecisive and confused • Lack of courage • Long-term fright becomes fear • Easily angered when startled
Fear	Kidney	• Involuntary urination (happens to children) • Depression • Unable to make decisions • Confused • Lack courage • Anxiety and agitation • Initially affects the heart but long term affects the kidney
Joy	Heart	• Feeling of agitation • Insomnia due to over stimulus • Palpitation • Unclear thinking • Heart attack

In the beginning of this section, I talked about how my 6 foot 5 inch colleague leaned over my work cubicle to harass me about "why I'm so happy." To be truthful, I wasn't happy after my ex-girlfriend and I separated. I was in total grief. But I knew how to manage my emotional energy.

Which organ does grief affect?

Right, the lungs...so I did the next simple and powerful qigong movement every day for thirty days, and at the end of thirty days, I found more peacefulness in my mind. Although I was sad that things didn't work out between us, I was able to move on with my life.

Do you know someone who tells you about his or her break up story over and over again? "I can't believe he cheated on me," said Amy, or "Why is this always happening to me?" said Mike, or "It's been three years since we broke up, and I can't seem to move up with my life. I'm so traumatized by love," said John, or "Why are men such assholes? Where are all the good men?" said Mary.

What happens when we continue to hold on to the heartbreaking experiences and relive our breakup stories over and over again? We allow our past experiences to dictate our future, and we'll never find the love that we deserve. Even if we did find another lover, eventually mistrust would kick in, and that relationship would fail too.

We try so hard to protect our hearts from getting hurt again, but when we build a wall to protect ourselves from another heartbreaking experience, who do we block out? We block out the bad guys, right? But at the same time, we block out the good guys.

For thirty days, I did qigong to open up my lungs, as I said, and I repeated a few powerful mantras. I did this five minute sequence every day, which I'm about to teach you, and I was able to tear down my own Berlin wall and moved on with my life.

ACTION STEP EXERCISES

Now's the time to take action. If you haven't downloaded your workbook yet ask yourself what's stopping you? Get this handled now.
Go to **www.AllanTing.com/IEMBookBonuses**

Advanced Energy Exercise
(refer to Energy Rich Workbook)

Exercise a: Frustration Release Meditation

CHAPTER 14

The Science of Being Thankful and Grateful

*"Trade your expectations for appreciation and
your whole world changes in an instant."*

— Tony Robbins

If you were to ask me what is the best secret sauce to have more happiness and energy in our lives, it would be cultivating thankfulness more consistently. One might say, "I hate my life, and I have nothing to be grateful about. Bad things always happen to me, and I have the worst luck ever!" While it might seem true in that person's mind, the reality is that it is his perception.

We can always find something to be thankful about, because there always will be someone in a worse situation than us. If you haven't seen the award winning documentary, *The Lost Boys of Sudan*, I suggest you watch it to give you some perspective. During Sudan's brutal, twenty-year civil war, more than 2.5 million people were killed and millions more scattered. More than twenty thousand boys and girls became orphaned. Does that give us a new perspective on how bad our lives are? Even if we are homeless, our lives are still much better than those in this film, because there are homeless shelters we can turn to for help.

Dr. P. Murali Doraiswamy, head of the division of biologic psychology at Duke University Medical Center said, "If [thankfulness] were a drug, it would be the world's best-selling product with a health maintenance indication for every major organ system." When we sincerely appreciate and feel thankful, our brain fires off several reward chemicals called dopamine and serotonin, neurotransmitters that make us feel blissful and peaceful, and oxytocin, the love hormone.

Here is what is interesting about these studies. Turns out that our brains can't tell the difference between reality and perceived reality. "...Many good and bad things happen in our life every day, but until they come to our own attention, we don't get the neurotransmitter release that allows us to feel good or bad," said Mitch Wasden, CEO of Ochsner Medical Center.

Wait, I'm confused. What does that mean? Does that mean we can influence our own thoughts and behavior if we became more aware with our thoughts? Yes, this explains why people feel all spectrums of emotions when they watch movies. Have you ever felt emotionally touched when you watched the romantic movie, *The Notebook?* Did you cringe and feel anxious when you watched *The Lord of The Rings* series? Did you feel lighthearted after watching the Oscar Award nominated Disney movie Up?

The movies, *The Notebook, The Lord of the Rings,* and *Up* are all fictional, yet we feel a wide spectrum of emotions watching them. Our brains aren't capable of deciphering what is real and what is not. *How happy we are has a direct response with the meaning that we put behind it.* It's whatever we focus on that creates the experience. Even if something great happened in our lives, we would always feel bitter, jaded, and robbed if we chose to focus on the negatives.

Let me share a story about a homeless man I encountered who chose to see the negativities in the world even when there was so much to be thankful and grateful for. A few years ago, I traveled to Washington DC for work. During the weekends, I did some sightseeing and wandered from The Natural History Museum to the Smithsonian Museums. When my stomach started growling, I decided to take a break for lunch. I walked towards Chinatown on H Street NW. As I pondered what food I wanted to eat, I saw a homeless man wearing a worn out, dirty, brown sports coat; a pair of greasy looking corduroy pants; and a pair of dress shoes that was once black but had turned gray. It seemed that he hadn't showered in days, with his strong body, uncombed hair, and shaggy beard.

While he was digging through the garbage bin, I walked up to the fifty-something-year-old man and asked him if he would like some food. "Hey, Mister. Are you hungry? Would you like me to buy you some food?" I questioned.

He looked at me with his weary brown eyes, nodded his head, and said, "Yes, I would like to eat."

I said, "Come with me," and he grabbed all of his belongings and a black carry-on suitcase with his left hand.

We walked into the nearest restaurant, which was Zengo, an upscale Latin/Asian fusion restaurant. I thought to myself, "Man, is he in luck today. He gets to eat gourmet food, not your Mickey D Big Mac."

I approached the well-dressed host wearing a black tailored suit, and explained the situation with the homeless man getting some food. I said, "Sir, I would like to get something to go for this gentleman. He is starving, and I'd like to give him some food."

The spiffy looking host looked at me, turned and looked at the dirty man with the brown jacket, and said, "You need to leave." He repeated again, "You need to leave *right now.*"

I looked at the host straight in the eyes and said, "I'm sorry to put you in this awkward position with the homeless man in the restaurant. I'd just like to get him some food and leave. The man is hungry, and I'm just doing him a favor so that he can pay it forward later when he gets back on his feet."

The host looked at him in disgust as he repeated again, "He needs to leave here."

I looked at the homeless man and said, "Sir, would you mind stepping outside for a moment while we order your food?"

Just then, the homeless man's personality came out, and he became Mr. Agro. He scolded the host at the top of his lungs, "You don't give a shit about if I live or not. I'm dying here. You don't give a shit that I'm dying. You don't care."

The angry man looked down towards the fancy carpet and mumbled, "No one cares about me, and I might as well be dead!" I was a bit thrown off with this situation, because I had fed many homeless people over the years, and never had I experienced something like this. One, it put me in a bad situation with the host, because I had brought the torn, brown jacketed man into the restaurant. I was somewhat responsible for this commotion. Second, he said, "No one cares about me. I'm dying here..." I was buying him food out of compassion and asking for nothing in return, and he still thought, "No one cares."

Instead of making the drama worse, I asked the homeless man politely, "Would you kindly please stand outside the door while I'm ordering your food?"

Looking disgusted, the homeless man dragged his beat up black suitcase and angrily walked outside the door.

As I waited for his food, the host found some compassion for the guy and said, "Let me get him a large sized Coke on the house." I thanked the host for his generosity and patience when he handed me the to-go bag and large drink. Then I walked outside of the restaurant and handed the food to the bitter homeless man and walked off in search for my food.

As I sat in a nearby Chinese restaurant ordering my food, I reflected on what had happened, because I'm a student of human behavior. I want to understand why people act the way they do. Some homeless people I've fed were very gracious and appreciative, and then there was Mr. Agro.

I also reflected back on my life when I was almost homeless twelve years ago, and I too was angry. But I learned to appreciate and be thankful for what I had. Today, I am appreciative of my good health and that I have a very loving family.

Perhaps if Mr. Agro had refocused his energy to be more thankful and appreciative, he would have stopped being so angry and taken a moment to see what was offered in front of him, which was a warm meal from a four star restaurant—instead of eating rotten leftover food from the garbage can. In addition, the resentful homeless man was not handicapped. He was capable of walking and digging his hands through garbage. He was not disfigured or an amputee. He was not a mute; he spoke perfectly. He was not blind and could see perfectly. Those things were a blessing and a miracle, if he could choose to see them that way. Instead, he played the victim role and blamed everyone else for his horrible life.

What this really boils down to is that we all have a choice. We have a choice to be grateful and thankful. Dalai Lama said, "When we meet real tragedy in life, we can react in two ways— either by losing hope and falling into self-destructive habits, or by using the challenge to find our inner strength..." If we consciously build our grateful and thankful emotional muscles, our lives will change before us—just like I took my life from near homelessness to where I am today. Everyone is capable of doing this, no matter what they have gone through in life.

CHAPTER 15

Emotional Detox and Cleansing Through Sound and Vibrations

"The sound body is the product of the sound mind."
— George Bernard Shaw

When George Bernard Shaw came up with his quote, he most likely meant a *sound mind* as having the capacity to think, reason, and understand oneself. He probably didn't think the actual vibration of the sound affected our organs as well.

We can tune and cleanse our organs through sound vibrations. Remember, different organs hold different emotions.

Now you're probably saying, "What the crap is this New Age stuff about vibrations?" Before you discount this practice, let's go back to something that is common sense but not common knowledge. Remember the "a-ha" moment we introduced in the beginning of this section, wherein we have epiphany moments and become really passionate? Turns out that "ha" is the cleansing sound for the heart in qigong. Are you still skeptical? The next time you yawn, pay attention to what's at the end. What sound do you make when yawn? Is there a "ah" or "ha" in the end of your breath?

How about when you laugh? What sound do you make? *Ha!* Got you! No pun intended. Why do people all around the world make the sound "ha" when they laugh? Sound vibration has been practiced since the fifth century in China, so if you say this is *"New Age,"* I would say this is really an *"Old School"* practice.

Does that mean we have to hear something funny before we make the sound "ha," or we have to yawn to make "ha" happen? It's not the chicken or the egg dilemma. We can govern our emotions by proactively cleansing our organs with sounds. As I've said, we clean out our wastebasket when it gets full, so why not clear our emotional garbage as well? Oh, by the way, what percentage of our bodies did we say are made of water? More than 80 percent, right? And what happens when sound vibrates through water? It creates a ripple, wave like effect, doesn't it? Remember the scene from *Jurassic Park* where the kids were in the Jeep looking at concentric circles in a cup of water as the T Rex approached them? Steven Spielberg used guitar strings and plucked them underneath the cup to achieve that vibrating effect, and we similarly can use sound to vibrate our body.

How many sounds are there?

Qigong practitioners use six healing sounds to clear, release, and purge our organs and tissues of bad, excess, and stagnant energy. There are six specific tones to open up our organs and help us release our negative emotions before adding fresh energy into our bodies.

The cardinal rule for effective sound vibration therapy is that we can feel the sound vibrating the targeted organs. It does take a little bit of practice, but one can easily feel the vibrations. Those vibrations help shake loose any toxic energy and emotional debris. In addition, practice with your eyes open, because if too much focus is internal, the bad energy or qi has a harder time leaving your body.

Do the six organ cleansing sounds (following) in order, and it is paramount that your breath should be smooth and even. If you have to grasp for a big inhale, you have over extended your breath.

It is very important to *remember that nothing is forced during breath work.*

Ready to do detox, do some spring-cleaning and release the negative emotions? Would you not ever empty the garbage in your house? Of course not! It's the same with our emotions. We collect emotional garbage and needs some emotional cleanse from time to time.

Head over towards your *Energy Rich Workbook and flip over to Advanced Emotional Detox Sound Cleansing Exercises* under Secret Energy Hack Section IV – Advanced Energy State: The Joy of Pure Energy. Learn how to emotionally detox and balance your body to cleanse out:

a. Frustration and anger
b. Insomnia and agitation
c. Burnout and exhaustion
d. Worry, anxiety and sadness
e. Fear and uncertainty

ACTION STEP EXERCISES

Want to get free updates and high performance training videos? Go now if you haven't already done so:
www.AllanTing.com/IEMBookBonuses

Advanced Energy Sound Cleansing Exercises
(refer to Energy Rich Workbook):

A. *Liver Cleanse – Anger and Frustration Release*

B. *Heart Cleanse – Agitation and Insomnia Release*

C. *Spleen Stomach – Burnout and Exhaustion Release*

D. *Lung – Worry, Anxiety and Sadness Release*

E. *Kidneys – Fear and Uncertainty Release*

F. *Harmonizing the Triple Burners Cleanse – Sound Body Balance Technique*

SECTION IV

Game Changer Questions

1. What were the top three things that you learned in this section, and if you applied them in my life consistently, how would you be able to focus even more at work?
2. If you were to adopt an even more powerful new identity or belief about yourself, who would you be? (Give your new identity a name, so that you can access this emotion anytime you want.)
3. If you're going to experience even more happiness in your life, what would you have to...?

There is one last advanced posture that I want to share with you. I'd love to invite you do this on a regular basis, because *success does not build on failure. Success only builds on success.*

So bring your right hand out, palm facing up. Reach your right hand to the sky. Bend your right elbow, and pat yourself on the back for your consistent effort.

Remember, *"No one can be your own best cheerleader but yourself. So be your own best cheerleader."*

We have covered a lot of ground in the last few sections, and I want to take a moment to honor you for following through. I want to take a moment and honor your hard work and commitment sticking it through with me. I'm also going to make living your high performance life even easier. I'll give you the abbreviated version of the exercises and a suggested routine so that you can start building your own consistent practice. Keep up the hard work, and we'll talk more in the next section.

Putting It All Together

"There is one thing that 99 percent of 'failures' and 'successful' folks have in common—they all hate doing the same things. The difference is successful people do them anyway. Change is hard. That's why people don't transform their bad habits, and why so many end up unhappy and unhealthy."

— Darren Hardy

Statistics have shown that more than 90 percent of people who bought a book never read past the first chapter. You are in the top percentile, and I want to congratulate you for sticking through it with me. I also want to honor your commitment for getting this far.

I don't say this lightly, because I believe you and I are kindred souls on this journey and became good friends along the way. I also believe that it's no accident that you and I have connected.

There is an old saying, "When the student is ready, the teacher will appear," and I want to thank you for allowing me to be your guide. It's an honor serving you. Deep down in my heart, it is my wish for you to continue consistently practicing what you have learned in this book. I look forward meeting you in person, and I can't wait to hear how your life has transformed.

To help you continue with your journey, I have put together an abbreviated version of the main concepts in this book to help guide your practice in your *Energy Rich Workbook* under Summary of All

Exercises. Here is the link to the *Energy Rich Workbook* if you happen to misplace your file. **www.AllanTing.com/IEMBookBonuses**

I understand you may have a busy schedule, so I have put together a framework to help you. The duration of the exercises are suggested. You can always modify the duration and mix and match the sequence to meet your emotional state and busy schedule.

Epilogue

"Kindness is more important than wisdom, and the recognition of this is the beginning of wisdom."

— Theodore Isaac Rubin

I have a core belief that if I were to learn anything, I would want to learn the core element—the essence of the material—because that is the 20 percent that will make the 80 percent impact in my life. When I started my journey into learning about energy, I sought out the direct source by asking a simple question, "How do I naturally get sustainable, massive energy with a small amount of effort and time." Through that question, I have gained a ferocious appetite for learning and trying different things.

I used to ask my teachers, "Why do we feel better after yoga and qigong classes?" and no one was able to give me a straight answer.

They would say, "You're letting go of anger," or, "You are opening up your body." No one could give me a definitive answer, but I wanted to replicate that experience to make my own practice more effective.

It wasn't until I combined my energy practice with neuroscience that I understood the alchemy of how to create massive energy. Just like an alchemist transforms lead into gold, I realized that if I mixed breathing, a change in posture, and other key elements, I was able to unlock my own energy.

I wanted to share my message and help people with chronic stress and fatigue to get out of their proverbial cages. I found the key to help them live better lives, so I started teaching.

Often, new students would approach me after class and ask me, "Where and who did you study with? Why is your teaching so different? Where can I study more of what you have taught?"

Usually my regular students would help me answer, "It's an Allan Ting method."

For years, my students have been asking me when my book and DVD are coming out. For years, I have been pushing them off, because writing is not my thing; English is my second language.

And I wanted to take a moment to thank and acknowledge my students for encouraging me to put my teachings in writing so that I can help even more people. I still have nightmares about my tenth grade high school English teacher lecturing me in front of the entire class for more than ten minutes. She asked me to stand right next to the podium with her while she drew red lines and circles on my term paper. When I got to college, a professor said to me at the end of my freshman year, "I'm passing you with a C, but you really need to take English 114 over again to build your foundation."

Have you ever been reluctant to do something like singing, playing a musical instrument, or even playing sports, because someone along the way told you that you were bad at it? That was me. I have been reluctant to write because of those nightmares. But for years, I wanted to write a book, because I wanted to share with everyone what I have learned.

But something happened in my life. Towards the end of 2011, my entire life fell apart. My career at a high tech company was in limbo, because I was burned out. I had travelled so much for work that I logged seventy-five hotel night stays in a year. That's almost three months of living out of a suitcase. My relationship suffered. My fiancé called it quits and we broke up.

As a man, I can count the number of times when I broke down and cried uncontrollably with only one hand because I really cared and loved her. I was crying my eyes out as she dropped me off at Los Angeles International Airport.

I said to myself, "Be strong, Allan. Things will get better. Just get through today, and tomorrow is another day." I told myself that over and over again to help get myself through that day.

Did you ever ask yourself these questions after a serious breakup? I mean questions like, "Where did our relationship go wrong? Have I done my best and given her everything?" These were the ones I asked myself.

When I sat down and meditated, the answers revealed right in front of me, as my inner voice said, "You have given your all, and you have done your best. You gave her everything and did all you could have. That is something you should be proud of."

But I was still really torn. I was really broken.

My heart was in pieces as I left LAX, wearing a pair of sunglasses at night for the first time. I didn't want the world to see me like this—weak and fragile.

I was free falling towards depression, and I knew I needed to somehow pick myself up quickly, because I support my mom and dad and had a hectic corporate job. I somehow needed to stop the bleeding, so the very next day, I dragged myself to a yoga class to move my body and start pushing the negative emotional toxins out of my body. Although I felt physically better after class, I knew my heart was still mangled in pieces.

You know when you go through a breakup, mixed emotions come up, and they get wrapped up into a continuous loop? Throughout the day, I felt many heavy emotions—from getting really pissed off, to wanting her back in my life, to wondering what I did wrong, to blaming her for why we didn't work out. My emotions were trapped inside this crazy figure eight loop, going from sadness to anger, anger to sadness, over and over in my head.

The worst part was that I still had to work fourteen hour days and on weekends to catch up. Heck, I even had to work during Thanksgiving and the day before Christmas writing statements of work. By January, I was burned out with my super stressful job. I asked my manager if I could take a sabbatical from work, and he gracefully supported my decision.

I felt like I had to get away from everything, so that I could have a better perspective. I took that opportunity and traveled so that I could pick up the pieces of my heart and get away from ever piling emails.

Within a few weeks, I booked a one-way ticket and went traveling around the world. My first stop was at Savusavu in Fiji for a nine day retreat. When I left SFO on Air Pacific heading for Fiji, I thought about doing a human experiment. As much as I was in pain, I decided I was going to implement everything that I had learned about human behavior, psychology, neuroscience, and high performance—and put it all into practice. I already knew the ingredients. I just needed to be my own alchemist and mix the formula together.

Even though I was suffering in deep depression and burnt out, I could have easily blamed people who had hurt me—focusing on how they had screwed up my life. This is something we could all easily do playing a "poor me" victim role.

Instead, I took a different approach. I committed myself to helping people who came across my path, despite how much pain I was in. In re-jogging my mental notes, I remembered that there are seven power formulas to getting unchained from depression.

For the sake of not turning this book into a five hundred pages novel, I will share with you the first teaching that completely transformed my life. Perhaps that will become the topic of my next book, as I continue on this journey.

1) Serve Others From Your Heart

When I arrived at the retreat in Fiji, I asked the facilitator if I could volunteer teaching yoga and qigong to the participants in the morning. I knew I had this gift, and was happy to serve others. He agreed, and I taught my classes from 7:30 am to 8:30 am in the morning.

On the eighth day of class, a young, dark haired young woman pulled me aside after class. She said, "Allan, I want to really thank you for teaching your energy classes every morning. Before I came to Fiji, I was really depressed. I even thought about committing suicide. The only reason I didn't was because I have three beautiful little girls. After taking your class, I'm no longer depressed, and I really want to thank you."

I met many random people who simply needed someone to listen to, and I was there to help support them.

In 2012, I met and served:

- A dog trainer who lost her dog—her best friend—and found equanimity.
- A man whose parents looked down on what he loved to do in life; I helped him find his passion.
- A dad who was overwhelmed with his job—and reconnected with what was important in his life: his beautiful wife and daughter.
- A father who beat his wife because he felt trapped and angry—and found his inner peace.
- A yoga teacher who overcame her self-doubt.
- A woman who overcame her depression after a divorce.

- A woman who finally forgave her deceased brother after more than twenty years.
- And many others.

The reason I'm sharing this with you is because often when we get hurt, we put up proverbial walls—thinking that we are protecting ourselves from getting hurt again. But in reality, as I mentioned in the book, when we block out the bad people, who do we also block out? We block out the good people coming into our lives don't we?

If I were to ask you, "Have you ever been heartbroken in your life before?" you would absolutely say, "Yes," wouldn't you? We all have experienced pain or trauma, and we all have been heartbroken before. This is a part of the human experience.

And learning to forgive and appreciate is also part of the human experience—the *learning* part.

Here is my message to you and the lesson that I learned from the hard breakup: the profound experience that I learned from serving others is that I saw bits and pieces of myself in everyone I had helped. Those bits and pieces ended up healing my heart and pain. I was no longer depressed, and I was able to forgive and let go of my anger, resentment, and depression.

The best part of this journey was that I met a young man whose passion was to spread love and joy. I learned that his mission in life was to inspire others to spread love and joy to their families, loved ones, friends, and even random strangers.

I don't know where you are in life right now—whether you are having the time of your time celebrating success or you are in a rut and a bit down in your luck. I do know this: *if you want to live a life of full joy and fulfillment, challenge yourself by serving others from your heart.*

The world needs us more than ever. One in every ten Americans is depressed. Those who are depressed also have higher rates of obesity, heart disease, stroke, sleep disorders, and are uneducated and have little access to medical insurance.

Do you know someone who is taking anti-depressants and is still depressed? Achieving a better life through chemistry alone isn't really working, is it?

My challenge to you is to share with people around you with the knowledge that you now possess. Even if your action were just as simple as a smile or a "thank you" to a random stranger at the grocery checkout line, it would brighten someone's day. When you smile, your body forces you to change your posture, doesn't it?

By working together, we can make a difference in the world, one person at a time. And together, we create this kindness ripple effect, like dropping a small pebble that releases small, spreading waves across the pond.

I found that young man in my heart. By serving the amazing people who I have met, and by giving them my unconditional love, I was able to help heal my heart in return. That year, I found what I was made of.

Within half a year, an amazing and beautiful woman came into my life, because *I stopped chasing love. I started doing what I love.*

Recently, I asked her why she fell in love with me, and she said, "I love how you're so passionate about your mission, and you know where you want to be. You inspire me to see a higher purpose in life. You want to serve people for the greater good."

I told her, "I believe everyone on this earth has his or her own mission to fulfill—some big and some small—but we are all equally important in how the world works."

I further said, "I know my passion has been to do philanthropy work ever since I was a kid. My mission in life is to train next generations of leaders by building schools in developing countries, so that kids can grow up leading their communities."

Now we're married, and we also have a newborn daughter. None of this would have happened if I had not dug deeply into my soul to find out what was my passion in life.

It is my sincere wish that you have found many "a-ha" moments and "golden nuggets" in this book. I ask that you apply what you have learned here, and I can't wait to hear from you about what life is like afterwards.

Challenge yourself by helping others, and see how your life changes right in front of you—because the fastest way out of depression is contribution. Someone out there will always be less fortunate than you are, and you will appreciate what you have just that much more.

I also look forward to hearing about your journey out in the world and your stories of serving others who are in need. Again, I believe that it's no accident that we have crossed paths, and I would love to continue with our friendship.

I would like to invite you to keep in touch with me. If you haven't already signed up for my updates on living a high performance life, enter your name and email at **www.AllanTing.com/IEMBookBonuses** to get my updated free training blog post, videos, and emails.

I would also like to invite you to join my High Performance coaching program, helping you achieve your ultimate goals. I don't know where you are in life right now. You're probably not where I was; you're probably much further along in this journey. Maybe you're where I am now: super excited about your life and just looking for that extra edge with your career, mission in life—or with your body, relationship, or finances. You may be wondering, *how do I get to the next level?*

On the other hand, maybe you're in a life transition. You are standing at a crossroad wondering which path to take, and your big concern is not knowing which is the right path. Because you don't want to make a big mistake, maybe you're stuck in the analysis paralysis phase, and this stress and your tension are building even more. You are asking: *What do I do? How do I move forward?*

The high performers in the world like Michael Jordan and Tony Robbins all had great coaches in their lives. And they know it is not the big things that change our lives, but it's the small changes coupled with consistent focus and consistent actions. It's the small shift that golfers do with their grip hold, the small tweak in angle, that helps them hit straighter and develop a longer drive.

Wherever you are right now in life, together you and I will help you find your sweet spot, because my passion is to serve you with my heart.

If things are going great in your career, you may know your kids are not getting enough attention, and you feel bad for not spending more time with them. It may be that you have a great relationship with your children, but you don't have time to take care of your body. You may take care of your body, but you don't have much time with your spouse. That is the nature of life in the Twenty-first Century. Whatever we focus on, we get more of.

The coaching program is about showing you step-by-step strategies to help you close the gap between where you are now and where you want to be. Of course, this is not about my coaching program or me. It's about you—and about the best of you. I'm talking about the part of you that knows you are destined for more. You are destined for more greatness.

It's a twelve-week course to help you find the best in yourself from these five main segments: amplified and sustained levels of CLARITY, ENERGY, COURAGE, PRODUCTIVITY, and INFLUENCE. These are the five areas in which the best performers in the world outshine others. I can't wait to take you there. Within a short period of time, we're going to get your life to a whole other level.

Go to www.AllanTing.com/Coaching, and fill out your 5 minutes high performance questionnaire to help you start defining your absolute crystal clear vision and results that you want to achieve. Today is the day to take your life to a whole new level. This is your time!

If you are more interested in philanthropy work, and I piqued your interest about building schools in developing countries, and you would like to join me in exploring this, I'd love to hear from you as well.

Together, we make this world a better place, one person at a time.

Until then,
Live your dreams
Love every moment
Journey with your heart by spreading love and joy
To the light within you. To the light within me.

Allan

References

Preface

1. Arianna Huffington, *Thrive: The Third Metric to Redefining Success and Creating a Life of Well Being, Wisdom, and Wonder* (New York: Harmony, 2015), 99–100.

2. American Psychological Association and Harris Interactive "Stress in the Workplace," *American Psychological Association* (March 2011): 2, accessed April 10, 2015. https://www.apa.org/news/press/releases/phwa-survey-summary.pdf.

3. Accenture "Defining Success 2013 Global Research Results," Accenture (2013): 10, accessed April 10, 2015. http://www.accenture.com/SiteCollectionDocuments/PDF/Accenture-IWD-2013-Research-Deck-022013.pdf.

4. "Starbucks Financial Statements," accessed January 23, 2015. http://www.bloomberg.com/research/stocks/financials/financials.asp?ticker=SBUX.

5. "Starbucks Annual Report," Starbucks Corp, accessed January 23, 2015. http://investing.businessweek.com/research/stocks/financials/financials.asp?ticker=SBUX

6. "Forbes.com," last modified February 8, 2012. http://www.forbes.com/sites/clareoconnor/2012/02/08/manoj-bhargava-the-mystery-monk-making-billions-with-5-hour-energy.

7. "The Mystery Monk Making Millions With 5-Hour Energy," *Living Essentials,* accessed January 25, 2015. http://www.forbes.com/sites/clareoconnor/2012/02/08/manoj-bhargava-the-mystery-monk-making-billions-with-5-hour-energy.

8. "American Workers Spend $1,000 A Year On Coffee, $2,000 A Year On Lunch," *The Huffington Post,* January 20, 2012, accessed April 10, 2015, http://www.huffingtonpost.com/2012/01/20/american-workers-coffee-spending_n_1219579.html.

9. "American Workers Spend $1,000 A Year On Coffee, $2000 A Year On Lunch," *The Huffington Post*, January, 24, 2012, accessed April 10, 2015, http://www.huffingtonpost.com/2012/01/20/american-workers-coffee-spending_n_1219579.html.

10. "Insufficient Sleep Is a Public Health Epidemic," Center for Disease Control, accessed January 22, 2015, http://www.cdc.gov/features/dssleep.

11. Herbert Benson and William Proctor, *The Relaxation Revolution: The Science and Genetics of Mind Body Healing*. (Scribner 1 edition, June 21, 2011).

12. Laura Petrecca and Julie Snider, "Always Working Our all-mobile world is killing the desktop – and our personal lives," *USA Today*, March 7, 2013, front page, accessed January 22, 15, http://www.usatoday.com/story/news/nation/2013/03/06/mobile-workforce -all-work/1958673.

13. "Chronic Health Conditions Cost U.S. $84 Billion in Lost Productivity Study Finds" *Health Living Blog*, May 7, 2013, http://www.huffingtonpost.com/2013/05/07/chronic-health-conditions -lost-productivity-absenteeism-missed-work_n_3232438.html.

Intro

14. "Build Positive Team and Family Spirit," Zappos IP, Inc, accessed January 21, 2015, http://about.zappos.com/our-unique-culture/zappos-core-values/build -positive-team-and-family-spirit

15. Tony Robbins, *Money Master the Game: 7 Simple Steps to Financial Freedom*. (Simon & Schuster, November 18, 2014), 576–577.

16. Max Nisen, "Why Executive Burnout is Such a Huge Problem," *Business Insider*, May 8, 2013, http://www.businessinsider.com/ceo-burnout-is-a-growing-problem -2013-5.

17. Jennifer Robison, "Happiness is Love – and $75,000," *Gallup Business Journal*, accessed April 10, 2015, http://www.gallup.com/businessjournal/150671/happiness-is-love-and-75k.aspx

18. G. Belenky, S.C. Marcy, & J.A. Martin, "Debriefings and Battle Reconstructions Following Combat." *The Gulf War and Mental Health: A Comprehensive Guide*. (Westport, CT: Praeger, 1996).

19. M. Rosenbloom, E.V Sullivan and A. Pfefferbaum, "Using Magnetic Resonance Imaging and Diffusion Tensor Imaging to Assess Brain Damage in Alcoholics." *Alcohol Research & Health* 27(2): 146–152, 2003, accessed 4/10/2015, http://pubs.niaaa.nih.gov/publications/aa63/aa63.htm

Section I: Boost Energy

20. Amy J.C. Cuddy, Caroline A. Wilmuth, and Dana R. Carney. "The Benefit of Power Posing Before a High-Stakes Social Evaluation." Harvard Business School Working Paper, No. 13- 027, September 2012, accessed April 10, 2015, http://dash.harvard.edu/handle/1/9547823.

21. Dr. Alexis Carrel, "On the Permanent Life of Tissues outside of the Organism," *Journal of Experimental Medicine* 15 (1912): 516–28.

22. "Chronic Dehydration More Common Than You Think," CBS Miami, July 2, 2013, accessed April 10, 2015, http://miami.cbslocal.com/2013/07/02/chronic-dehydration-more-common -than-you-think.

23. F. Batmanghelidj, MD, *Your Body's Many Cries for Water,* Global Health Solutions, Inc.; third edition (November 1, 2008).

24. "Drinking Enough Water," WebMD, accessed January 25, 2013, http://www.webmd.com/a-to-z-guides/drinking-enough-water-topic-overview.

25. "Why Successful People Leave Early," *Business Insider,* May 4, 2011, accessed April 10, 2015, http://www.businessinsider.com/leave-work-early-2011-5#ixzz3PsA9kFjf.

Section II: Energy Drainers

26. Dr. George Nichopoulos, *The King and Dr. Nick: What Really Happened to Elvis and Me.* (Nashville, TN: Thomas Nelson, January 5, 2010).

27. Christopher Bergland, January 22, 2013, "Cortisol: Why "The Stress Hormone" Is Public Enemy No. 1?" *Psychology Today,* January 22, 2013, accessed April 20, 2015, http://www.psychologytoday.com/blog/the-athletes-way/201301/ cortisol-why-the-stress-hormone-is-public-enemy-no-1

28. Ross McLennan, *Booze, Bucks, Bamboozle, & You!* (Sane Press, 1978).

29. Erica Goode, "Power of Positive Thinking May Have a Health Benefit, Study Says," The *New York Times,* September 2, 2013, accessed April 10, 2015, http://www.nytimes.com/2003/09/02/health/power-of-positive-thinking -may-have-a-health-benefit-study-says.html

Section III: Manage Energy For Life

30. "Dr. Oz on Using Qigong to Combat Aging Video," Harpo Production, accessed January 31, 2015,
    http://www.oprah.com/health/Dr-Oz-in-Using-qigong-to-Combat-Aging-Video

31. GoChi, H. Amagase and D.M. Nance, "A Randomized, Double-blind, Placebo-controlled, Clinical Study of the General Effects of a Standardized Lycium Barbarum (Goji) Juice," *The Journal of Alternative and Complementary Medicine*," May 2008.

32. Tamara Hoffman, MD, "Ginger: An Ancient Remedy and Modern Miracle Drug." *Hawai'i Medical Journal* (2007), Volume 66, No. 12, accessed January 31, 2015,
    http://hjmph.org/HMJ_Dec07.pdf

33. "Coconut Water is an Excellent Sports Drink—for Light Exercise," American Chemical Society, release August 20, 2012, accessed April 10, 2015,
    http://www.acs.org/content/acs/en/pressroom/newsreleases/2012/august/coconut-water-is-an-excellent-sports-drink-for-light-exercise.html

34. "The Surprising Health Benefits of Coconut Oil," doctoroz.com, accessed February 1, 2015,
    http://www.doctoroz.com/article/surprising-health-benefits-coconut-oil?page=1.

35. López Ledesma R, Frati Munari AC, Hernández Domínguez BC, Cervantes Montalvo S, Hernández Luna MH, Juárez C and Morán Lira S, "Monounsaturated Fatty Acid (Avocado) Rich Diet for Mild Hypercholesterolemia." *Archives of Medical Research* 1996 Winter; 27(4): 519-23. Abstract.

36. Victor L Fulgoni, Mark Dreher and Adrienne J Davenport, "Avocado Consumption Is Associated with Better Diet Quality and Nutrient Intake, and Lower Metabolic Syndrome Risk in US Adults: Results from the National Health and Nutrition Examination Survey (NHANES) 2001–2008," *Nutrition Journal.* January 2, 2013.

37. Ding H, Chin YW, Kinghorn AD and D'Ambrosio SM, "Chemopreventive Characteristics of Avocado Fruit," *Seminars in Cancer Biology.* 2007 Oct, 17(5):386-94.

38. Boileau C, Martel-Pelletier J and Caron J et al, "Protective Effects of Total Fraction of Avocado/Soybean Unsaponifiables on the Structural Changes in Experimental Dog Osteoarthritis: Inhibition of Nitric Oxide Synthase and Matrix Metalloproteinase-1." *Arthritis Research & Therapy*. Epub Mar 16, 2009.

Section IV: Advanced Energy State: The Joy of Pure Energy

39. Arianna Huffington, "Arianna Huffington on Burning Out at Work, "Bloomberg Business, March 14, 2013, accessed April 10, 2015, http://www.bloomberg.com/bw/articles/2013-03-14/arianna-huffington -on-burning-out-at-work

40. Leslie Kwoh, "When the CEO Burns Out, " *Wall Street Journal*, May 7, 2013, accessed April 10, 2015, http://www.wsj.com/articles/SB1000142412788732368760457846912 4008524696

41. Harry Levinson, "When the CEO Burns Out," *Harvard Business Review*, July 1996, accessed April 10, 2015, https://hbr.org/1996/07/when-executives-burnout/ar/1

42. Connie Guglielmo, "Mobile Traffic Will Continue To Rise, Rise, Rise As Smart Devices Take Over The World, " *Forbes*, February 5, 2014, http://www.forbes.com/sites/connieguglielmo/2014/02/05/mobile -traffic-will-continue-to-rise-rise-rise-as-smart-devices-take-over-the-world/

43. Andrew Lipsman, "Major Mobile Milestones in May: Apps Now Drive Half of All Time Spent on Digital," June 25, 2014, acccessed April 10, 2015, http://www.comscore.com/Insights/Blog/Major-Mobile-Milestones-in -May-Apps-Now-Drive-Half-of-All-Time-Spent-on-Digital

44. "Insufficient Sleep Is a Public Health Epidemic," Center for Disease Control, accessed January 13, 2015, http://www.cdc.gov/features/dssleep.

45. Stephanie Schupska, "Not Enough Sleep: 7 Serious Health Risks," WebMD, October 5, 2010, http://www.webmd.com/sleep-disorders/features/not-enough-sleep-7 -serious-health-risks

46. Carolyn Gregoire, "This Is The New Favorite Pastime Of The Business Elite (Hint: It's Not Golf)," *Huffington Post*, September 18, 2013, accessed April 10, 2015, http://www.huffingtonpost.com/2013/09/18/leaders-meditation_n _3916003.html

47. Katie Little, "Severe Ski Accident Spurs Aetna CEO to Bring Yoga to Work," CNBC.com, March 19, 2013, accessed April 10, 2015, http://www.cnbc.com/id/100569740#.

48. Sue McGreevey, "Eight Weeks to a Better Brain," *Harvard Gazette,* January 21, 2011, accessed April 10, 2015, http://news.harvard.edu/gazette/story/2011/01/eight-weeks-to-a-better-brain/

49. Richard J. Davidson and Antoine Lutz, "Buddha's Brain: Neuroplasticity, and Meditation," *IEEE Signal Process Magazine.* January 1, 2008, 25(1): 176–174. PMCID: PMC2944261 http://www.ncbi.nlm.nih.gov/pmc/articles/PMC2944261/ NIHMSID: NIHMS83558

50. "Demystifying Meditation—Brain Imaging Illustrates How Meditation Reduces Pain," Wake Forest Baptist Medical Center, last updated. January 20, 2013, accessed April 10, 2015, http://www.wakehealth.edu/News-Releases/2011/Demystifying_Meditation_Brain_Imaging_Illustrates_How_Meditation_Reduces_Pain.htm

51. Clifton B. Parker, "Stanford Scholar Helps Veterans Recover from War Trauma," *Stanford Report,* September 5, 2014, accessed April 10, 2015, http://news.stanford.edu/news/2014/september/meditation-helps-ptsd -090514.html

52. Eileen Luders, Florian Kurth, Emeran A. Mayer, Arthur W. Toga, Katherine L. Narr and Christian Gaser, "The Unique Brain Anatomy of Meditation Practitioners: Alterations in Cortical Gyrification," *Frontiers in Human Neuroscience,* February 29, 2012.

53. Michael Gershon, *The Second Brain: A Groundbreaking New Understanding of Nervous Disorders of the Stomach and Intestine.* (Harper Perennial, November 17, 1999).

54. Mikaela Conley, "Thankfulness Linked to Positive Changes in Brain and Body," *Good Morning America,* November 23, 2011, accessed April 10, 2015, http://abcnews.go.com/Health/science-thankfulness/story?id=15008148.

Epilogue

55. "Unhappiness by the Numbers: 2012 Depression Statistics," *Healthline,* accessed Febuary 2, 2015, http://www.healthline.com/health/depression/statistics-infographic

About the Author

Allan Ting is a #1 International Best Selling Author, Professional Speaker and Certified High Performance Coach who has been invited to speak on ABC, NBC, CBS, Fox, and CW news.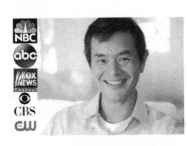

He is one of the top high performance trainers in the world and leads seminars and retreats in the US and Abroad. He has taught at large companies like Yahoo, HP, Amazon, eBay, Cisco, VMware, Microsoft, Motorola, and at Tony Robbins' live seminars.

Allan is a member of the Expert Industry Association, a Certified High Performance Coaches, Certified Advance Health NLP Coach, Certified Yoga Teacher and a part of Tony Robbins' Senior Leadership team.

Visit him and receive free training at
www.AllanTing.com/IEMBook.